UNE
JOY
and
SORROW

UNDERSTANDING JOY and SORROW

ACHARYA MAHAPRAGYA

TRANSLATORS
MUKHYA NIYOJIKA
SADHVI VISHRUT VIBHA
SADHVI VANDANASHREE

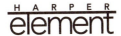

First published in India in 2012 by Element
an imprint of HarperCollins *Publishers* India
a joint venture with
The India Today Group

Copyright © Jain Vishva Bharati 2012

ISBN: 978-93-5029-391-1

2 4 6 8 10 9 7 5 3 1

Acharya Mahapragya asserts the moral right to be identified as the author of this work

All rights reserved. No part of this publication may be reproduced, stored in a retrieval system, or transmitted, in any form or by any means, electronic, mechanical, photocopying, recording or otherwise, without the prior permission of the publishers.

HarperCollins *Publishers*
A-53, Sector 57, Noida, Uttar Pradesh 201301, India
77-85 Fulham Palace Road, London W6 8JB, United Kingdom
Hazelton Lanes, 55 Avenue Road, Suite 2900, Toronto, Ontario M5R 3L2
and 1995 Markham Road, Scarborough, Ontario M1B 5M8, Canada
25 Ryde Road, Pymble, Sydney, NSW 2073, Australia
31 View Road, Glenfield, Auckland 10, New Zealand
10 East 53rd Street, New York NY 10022, USA

Typeset in 12/15 Adobe Caslon Pro by
R. Ajith Kumar

Printed and bound at
Thomson Press (India) Ltd

CONTENTS

Preface		vi
1.	Sorrow and the human mind	1
2.	Problems and sorrow: Two separate entities	9
3.	The invisible world	16
4.	Karma: The seeds of joy and sorrow	22
	Meditation: Antaryatra	29
5.	Desire: The root cause of sorrow	32
6.	Anger: The fire that burns happiness	40
7.	Can sorrow be reduced?	49
8.	Stress and sorrow	57
	Kayotsarga: Relaxation	64
9.	Freedom from sorrow	67
10.	Spiritual joy	73
11.	Self-realization: A step towards a happy life	83
12.	Who am I?	90
	Meditation: Perception of breathing	97
13.	Who is the happiest man?	100
14.	Happiness through contemplation	108

CONTENTS

15.	Joy lies within	115
16.	Equilibrium: The hidden secret of absolute happiness	122
	Meditation: Perception of the body	128
17.	Amity leads to happiness	133
18.	Standing alone in a crowd	139
19.	Happiness through detachment	147
20.	Achieving happiness by going beyond the mind	154
21.	Happiness and fearlessness	160
	Contemplation of fearlessness	170

PREFACE

I went to the market in Kolkata but I did not find any shop where joy was being sold.

I went to the market in Mumbai. I continued my search for a place where I could buy joy, but with no result.

I went to the market in Surat, the diamond city. There was no signboard indicating a place where joy was on sale.

I went to the market in Delhi, the capital of India. Not a single businessman did I find selling joy.

I could find no shops selling joy in any of the other metropolitan cities, such as Chennai or Bengaluru, either. There is no factory manufacturing it, nor has any high technology been discovered which can produce joy. Then, the question arises: From where does joy come? From where can it be obtained?

Long research has revealed that neither joy nor sorrow can be produced or sold in the market. Joy and sorrow are the rays of consciousness that cannot be created.

The cycle of joy and sorrow is perennial. A man is joyful sometimes and at other times, sorrowful. Favourable conditions stimulate joy, whereas unfavourable conditions result in sorrow.

The transformation of consciousness brings a change in the stimulation of joy and sorrow. A man with an enlightened consciousness remains calm and peaceful even in an adverse situation. A man with a dormant consciousness will remain tense and restless even in a favourable situation.

There are various causes that activate a feeling of joy or sorrow:

- Remembering joy or sorrow experienced in the past
- Imagining joy or sorrow
- Thinking of joy or sorrow

The theory of karma is a theory of subtle vibrations. Karma is the core of an individual's internal condition. Sometimes, we become sorrowful without any external cause; this happens because of the intense force of karmic waves.

SPIRITUAL SORROW

Spirituality means that whatever happens takes place in the innermost layers of consciousness. Negative emotions, like anger, pride and greed, lie in pure consciousness and are termed spiritual vices. Positive emotions, like forgiveness, modesty and contentment, which also lie in pure consciousness, are called spiritual virtues. Spiritual vices cause sorrow while spiritual virtues lead to happiness.

A person who has faith in the power of action and effort can transform sorrowful moments into moments of happiness through a positive attitude. On the other hand, a man whose consciousness is dormant, through his negative attitude, will transform a moment of joy into sorrow.

We may ask here, what exists in larger quantities in this world? Joy or sorrow? The common reply would be that this world is full of sorrow. A man always finds himself surrounded by problems.

I believe in the soul. I believe in the soul as the doer of everything. Therefore, a man himself is responsible for the joy and the sorrow he experiences.

In *Yoga Darshan* there is an explanation of the relation between sorrow and the fickleness of the mind. A steady mind can reduce a big incident to a small one. The less the fickleness, the less the sorrow. On the other hand, a man with an unsteady mind will magnify a small issue into a big one. The more the fickleness, the greater the sorrow.

Spirituality prescribes the following aphorisms to transform sorrow into happiness:

- The body and the soul are not identical. One who practises the science of the separation of body and soul transforms the consciousness of agony into the consciousness of bliss.
- Consciousness is free from all kinds of ailments. I reside in my consciousness. The disease occurs in the body and not in the consciousness. Therefore, I am not subjected to pain.

The sensation of sorrow can be reduced and terminated through the practice of meditation and contemplation.

The various aspects of sorrow and joy have been discussed in this book. Happiness and sorrow have been analysed in several of my books and lectures. Mukhya Niyojika Sadhvi Vishrut Vibhaji has selected some flowers of joy and sorrow from those books and lectures and, consequently, a beautiful garland has been woven. Sadhvi Vandanashree assisted her in this task.

PREFACE

The reader himself will reach the conclusion that joy is greater than sorrow. Joy is turned into sorrow by those whose world is confined to the materialistic approach. For such persons, there will always be more sorrow than joy.

The gist of this book is that a person should develop samyagdarshan–right vision and right attitude.

The translators deserve high praise for the good work done by them.

— **Acharya Mahapragya**

1
SORROW AND THE HUMAN MIND

We human beings are connected to a vast world of living organisms, of which we form a small part. Living beings can be classified into three categories which may be described as those who are:
- Devoid of a mind
- Endowed with a mind
- Beyond a mind

Worms, insects, flies and other similar creatures form the first category. There is no mental development in them and their life merely depends on physical consciousness. They can be termed as underdeveloped living beings.

Human beings fall into the second category. They are blessed with a wonderful brain which has the capacity to think, to imagine and to memorize. Using it, man has progressed from the Stone Age to the Atomic Age and is now heading towards the Nano Age.

UNDERSTANDING JOY AND SORROW

It is natural that where there is capacity to think, there will be different ideas; and where there are thoughts, there are bound to be conflicts. No mental activity is free from the clutches of conflict. Agony, struggle and depression are all by-products of the mind. Happiness and peace are the first priorities of a human being. Nobody really wants to be sad. Living beings which are devoid of a mind also suffer, but in the absence of mental activities, they are less expressive. The only pain they suffer is physical. A tree suffers pain when its leaves are plucked or its branches are broken, but this pain is momentary—it lasts only as long as the action lasts. Once the action stops, the pain disappears.

Such is not the case with humans. Humans are the smartest creatures in the world, but they are burdened with sorrow. If a man is injured, he feels unbearable pain which will last until it is cured. This physical pain is linked with the mind and it turns into a sensation. Because of his mental development, man leads a life full of sorrow. If he was lacking in a developed brain, he would not suffer from any kind of mental turmoil. The pain would stop with the end of the incident itself.

If a man is physically injured he experiences pain, but he may soon forget it. This may not be so when he is verbally abused. Because of a sharp memory, a powerful imagination and the capacity to think, a man tries to reason out everything and the matter does not come to an end. Man's habit of reacting and retaliating is inevitable, and looking for a solution to eradicate it cannot be analysed or explained. The more developed his mind, the greater is the sorrow in his life. Mental development has proved to be a boon as well as a curse to the human race. Unfortunately, this boon and this curse cannot be separated from each other.

Even for King Midas, who was blessed with the golden touch, the boon turned out to be a curse. His greed for gold made him lose his beloved daughter who, like his material possessions, turned into a golden statue. His happiness at attaining an immense amount of gold immediately turned into unbearable sorrow. Now, the question arises: can we protect ourselves from the curse of mental development? The afflictions of this age compel us to think that it would have been better for man to be devoid of a mind. But, having reached levels of development hitherto undreamt of, it is not reasonable to think so. It would be better to look for a solution to eradicate the issue of mental sorrow. The problem is, how can one reduce sorrow? Meditation is the answer to the problem. Mental development can continue to be a boon only if a person practises deep meditation. It can keep a man free from different kinds of sorrow. To reduce distress, one has to reach a state beyond the mind: a state of mental development where the normal mental process declines. This state of mind can be achieved only through meditation.

The third category of living beings includes those who have the capacity to go into a state beyond the mind. In this state, one is free of thoughts and imagination. There exists only light and pure consciousness, resulting in the end of misery and leading one to experience true joy.

When the mind is active, sorrow and negative emotions, like day and night, cannot be separated from each other. The state of the mind keeps on changing continuously. Sometimes it struggles with restlessness and at other times, it rests in peace.

Once, Prince Bhadrabahu, going through the city with his minister's son Sukeshi, noticed a crowd. The curious prince asked, 'Why have so many people gathered here?' Sukeshi answered, 'It is a cremation ground and a dead body is being cremated.'

UNDERSTANDING JOY AND SORROW

The ignorant prince asked, 'Why is the body being cremated? Why isn't it preserved?'

Sukeshi replied, 'When there is no life in the body, it rots and stinks. So it has to be cremated.'

The prince, who was very proud and fond of his beautiful body, asked, 'Will my body too be cremated one day?'

Sukeshi replied, 'Certainly, it will be.'

The realization of this truth made the prince furious. He was terrified by the idea of cremation. His pride in his body vanished, and he became sad and depressed. The king, who came to know the reason for his son's sadness, took him to a holy man and narrated the whole incident.

The holy man addressed the prince, 'False knowledge is making you sorrowful. This physical body is not real beauty. Real beauty resides within you in the form of consciousness. Try to perceive that.'

The prince realized the truth and his mind became calm and peaceful.

STATES OF MIND

There are three states of mind:
- Restless
- Peaceful
- Ecstatic

The human mind remains restless; rarely does it experience the true happiness that comes from tranquillity. The rich and the poor alike suffer from agitated states of mind. The poor are unhappy due to lack of resources and the rich, in spite of having abundant wealth, are never satisfied. It has been noticed that the rich people are more restless than the poor.

The human mind is in a state of rest when the owner's emotions are under control, but this state does not last long. Fickleness of mind makes a man continually restless.

The third state of mind occurs when one goes beyond the mind. This state can be experienced through meditation. Here, the mind remains inactive while the psyche becomes active. Mind and psyche are quite different from each other. What is the difference between them? All aspects of life cannot be explained on the basis of the mind only. It has its own limits while the psyche is quite comprehensive. A combined explanation of mind and psyche can draw a complete picture of behaviour and conduct. The mind can stop functioning but the psyche continues to perform. The activeness of the mind suppresses the psyche. When the mind is in a state of tranquillity—that is, when one goes beyond the mind—the psyche becomes active. Meditation is the means for triggering one's psyche. An over-active mind increases the sorrow within. In the state beyond the mind, sorrow comes to an end, whatever may be the cause of distress. The end of restlessness of the mind results in the absence of thoughts and distress.

Maharshi Patanjali described sorrow as the first consequence of an unsteady mind. The greater the fickleness, the greater is the sorrow. Nobody wants to suffer but it is unavoidable because man does not understand the fundamental cause of misery. The general perception is that unfavourable conditions cause sorrow. However, this is not enough to explain the degree of suffering one goes through because of these conditions. The amount of sorrow one experiences is practically immeasurable.

MEDITATION: NOT JUST A MENTAL EXERCISE
The only solution to overcome distress is to go into a state that is beyond the mind. The practical solution is meditation. The

objective of meditation is to go into a state beyond the mind and to realize the conscious mind. Its goal is not to gain control over one's mind. If we confine mediation to a mental level it will prove to be merely a mental exercise.

A herdsman used to work for a pandit. One day he asked for his salary for the month. The pandit said, 'You seem to be ignorant about the doctrine of Vedanta. According to it, each and every living entity is considered Brahma. And since everyone is identical to the next person, how can I pay you a salary?'

The herdsman was baffled by this behaviour. He went to his other employer and asked him for his salary. This employer replied, 'Don't you know the teachings of Lord Buddha? According to him, everything in this world is transitory. You are no longer the herdsman who grazed my cows and I am no longer the man whose cattle you took for grazing. In these circumstances, how can I pay you a salary?'

The herdsman was shocked. He felt confused and helpless. Finally, he approached a wise man for help. The wise man advised him, 'If the cows are still with you, don't return them tomorrow.' He then explained the plan to the herdsman.

The next day, the cows were not returned to their owners. The pandit rushed to the herdsman's place and inquired about his cattle. The herdsman said, 'Which cows are you asking about? Have you forgotten that the whole world is identical to "Brahma"? So how can I give you the cows and how can you take them? You may return to your home.'

The pandit realized his mistake. He immediately paid the herdsman his salary and took his cows.

The second employer also came to the herdsman and asked angrily, 'Where are my cows? Why have they not been returned yet?'

SORROW AND THE HUMAN MIND

The herdsman asked, 'Which cows? Whose cows? Everything has changed. The cows that are present are no longer the cows that had come for grazing. Go home and chant the mantras of transitivity.'

The employer realized that he was entangled in his own logical web and accepted his mistake. He immediately gave the herdsman his salary and took his cattle back.

This is an example of mental exercise. Philosophy too has been confined to being a mental puzzle. As long as the mental exercise and the philosophical puzzle continue, religion will not be able to express its true meaning, nor will the philosophers be able to reveal reality, which is the true aim of philosophy. In order to realize the truth, one has to go beyond the limits of the mind.

We are habituated to staying on the mental level round the clock. Even while sleeping, the mental activity does not stop. We should try to spend at least twenty to thirty minutes a day in the state which will take us into the state beyond the mind. This will open up a different horizon of experience which will, in turn, reveal a new way of life where the light of consciousness removes the darkness of mental activity.

To achieve this stage, initially one needs strong support. An infant, when learning to walk, requires his mother's support but when he grows up, he can walk independently. A boat is needed to cross a river. The practitioner of meditation should always keep in mind that support is essential but not everlasting. He should try to reach that state of meditation where no support is required and where he can enter a world that is free of all kinds of sorrow.

ESSENCE

- Living beings can be devoid of a mind, endowed with a mind or in a state beyond the mind.
- Man, because of his mental development, suffers from pain that lasts for a long time. His habit of reasoning out everything, remembering and retaliating creates a web of sorrow.
- Achieving a higher mental state, where one goes beyond the mind with the help of meditation, frees one from thought and imagination, and helps one experience a state of ecstasy.
- The mind can be in three different states: restless, at rest, or in ecstasy.
- The mind, because of its fickleness, swings between the restless and the restful states.
- The ecstatic state can be achieved through meditation which activates the psyche and ends the activities of the mind.
- Meditation should not remain a mere mental exercise because, then, it will not serve its main purpose.
- To achieve the ecstatic state, one may need support but one should not cling to it. One should practise meditation to reach a state where no support is required and one can enter the world free from all sorrows.

2
PROBLEMS AND SORROW: TWO SEPARATE ENTITIES

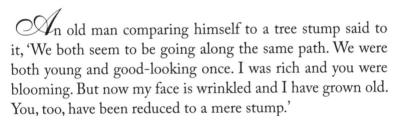

An old man comparing himself to a tree stump said to it, 'We both seem to be going along the same path. We were both young and good-looking once. I was rich and you were blooming. But now my face is wrinkled and I have grown old. You, too, have been reduced to a mere stump.'

The tree stump replied with a smile, 'I am not like you. I do not sing songs of sorrow. It is autumn now but once spring comes, I will regain my beauty. The hope of the coming spring keeps me happy, but you will continue to be sad.'

The tree stump and the old man are both in the same situation. But the man is full of sorrow while the tree stump is not. Why should this be so? Despite the similarity in the situation, there is a difference in the attitude, and we need to find out the reason.

SORROW AND THE SENSES

The experience of distress is different for every individual. Some magnify a small situation while others find comfort in treating situations lightly. Behaviour in a given situation distinguishes a prudent man from an over-sensitive one.

An over-sensitive person usually takes small and insignificant incidents to heart and it keeps him distressed. Even minor situations easily affect him. On the other hand, a wise man handles every situation, small or big, with a positive attitude and remains happy.

Knowledge is pure consciousness while sensations represent physical consciousness. A person who believes in physical consciousness is more sensitive and is apt to build a world of sorrows around himself. Such a person believes in and works only on the basis of the knowledge gained through the senses. Senses create an illusion because what they perceive is not always true. False perceptions create illusions and can be a major reason for sorrow.

Once a lion, the king of the jungle, had a wise jackal as his minister. Now, this jackal wielded a big influence over the king. Every creature in the jungle was jealous of him, and tried hard to get rid of him. They made a plot and managed to get the king's cook to help them. From the next day, the cook started to send only one-fifth of the regular quantity of meat to the king and the rest to the jackal. This continued for three days.

On the fourth day, the lion was furious and asked, 'Why has the quantity of my meat decreased?' The animals at court immediately blamed the jackal for the act. The lion visited the jackal's den, found a large amount of meat lying there, and decided to punish the jackal.

PROBLEMS AND SORROW: TWO SEPARATE ENTITIES

The mother lioness advised her son: 'Before you take any action, think over it. Everything you see is not always as it seems. The sky looks blue but it is not so. The glow-worm seems to be a small ball of fire but it is not. You should look for the truth in the matter before taking any action.' The lion decided to do so, and called for the jackal, and questioned him. The jackal replied, 'I was out for the past four days, I don't know who kept the meat there.' The lion realized his mistake and said that he would look into the matter.

JOY, SORROW AND THE SOUL

Sorrow exists; the cause of sorrow also exists. Joy exists, and so does the cause of joy. This is a universal truth, it cannot be denied. Unfavourable conditions and circumstances give rise to sorrow while favourable ones give rise to joy. Joy consists of three elements:

- The source or the ingredients of joy
- The sensation of joy
- The internal experience of the consciousness of joy

Similarly, there are three elements of sorrow:

- The ingredients of sorrow
- The sensation of sorrow
- The internal experience of the conciousness of sorrow

The soul in itself is free of sorrow, which is a sensation aroused by the material world. The real nature of the soul is joyful whereas sorrow is an imposed feature.

SORROW AND SUFFERING

Man cannot avoid sorrow, however much he tries. There are two main reasons for this:

- Habit
- The rise of asatavedaneya karma

A man may be enormously rich with all kinds of luxuries but he is still not happy. What makes him sorrowful? It could be the habit of negative thinking that compels him to lead a miserable life.

A man remembers harsh words spoken to him by his dead father years ago. Those memories still haunt him. This sorrow is due to no immediate reason, but merely a habit of remembering an unpleasant incident of the past. Another reason could be the rise of karma. When the fruition of previous karma occurs in the present life it gives rise to unfavourable situations. The fruition of karma is not a phenomenon related to the present birth, but to all the karma that one has accumulated through one's deeds in previous births.

Sorrow and problems are not the same. One person can create a problem but it is not necessary that it should make another sorrowful. This fact is revealed by many spiritual teachers. Ram was exiled for fourteen years, and he had to face countless difficulties for a long time, but that did not make him sorrowful.

Were the lives of Mahavira and Buddha devoid of obstacles? No, but those difficulties did not make them sorrowful. Acharya Bhikshu went through many adverse conditions but that did not discourage him. Even poison was not a cause for grief for Meera and Socrates.

These great persons are icons of wisdom. They lived their lives beyond physical consciousness, making it impossible for sorrow to even touch them. That is why they enjoyed unlimited happiness.

The concept of living beyond physical consciousness is spirituality. It means the development of extrasensory perception. In such a condition, neither habit nor karma can make one sorrowful.

For many, it is difficult to believe that even the greatest adversities are not capable of making a person sorrowful if he doesn't wish to be. A person of wisdom ignores problems and keeps sorrow at bay.

IDENTIFYING THE IDEAL

In order to attain such wisdom one has to set goals and practise meditation. The goal should be to uncover knowledge, bliss, power and the hidden virtues of the soul. 'Arhats', the enlightened souls, are at their supreme form and beyond sectarianism. They are the highest ideal. Whole-hearted devotion to one's goal leads a person to the state where he realizes the line of demarcation between the world of knowledge and the world of sensation. Only then he is enlightened with true knowledge.

One has to train the mind to develop imagination and will power. The purpose of this training is to enable the mind to see things clearly. Imagination gives a definite and clear form to our ideals. Bhavana, or suggestion through symbols, activates the will which motivates us to move towards the ideal we have set for ourselves.

Then, a man's resolution should be firm: 'I am totally dedicated to my ideal. There is no sensation of attachment or aversion, superiority or inferiority, but there is a flow of consciousness, of the eternal truth.' To experience total identification with the 'ideal' should be a man's real object. It was devotion to this object that made it possible for Socrates and Meera to drink without hesitation the poison given to them. Total dedication changes poison to nectar. A dedicated person can tolerate the most adverse circumstances and remain detached from them. In Patanjali's *Yoga Darshan*, it is known as samaapatit.

The simultaneous awakening of new consciousness keeps a person away from the sharp sting of sorrow. At this stage, the rise of karma may cause physical illness but cannot make a man sorrowful. Some people have the ability to bear physical pain and still have mental peace. They remain cheerful and affirm that they are in a state of perfect bliss. From where does this bliss come? In spite of being in a state of physical discomfort, they are happy because they have identified their ideal.

A religious man may feel as much sorrow as an irreligious man. It would be irrelevant to differentiate between them. It is understandable that an irreligious man should be subject to sorrow, but it might seem strange that a religious person becomes sorrowful too. Both are subjected to sorrow but the effect of sorrow on either individual depends on his internal state. A religious person understands that adversities are a part of human life, but an irreligious person cannot accept this fact and is apt to become sorrowful.

In this context, we should try to understand the definition of a religious person. One who isn't sorrowful under any circumstances is truly religious. Meditation is required to attain this state. Theory devoid of practice can never bring the desired result. By practising meditation, we can transform our consciousness from physical pleasure to eternal happiness. It will also help us live a life of wisdom and realize the absolute truth.

ESSENCE

- Knowledge gained through the senses is one of the major causes of sorrow.
- A negative attitude may develop illusions that can lead to sadness, while a positive attitude may change sadness to happiness.
- Sorrow may be the result of mere habit or of the friction of karmas, leading to sufferings.
- Living beyond the physical consciousness helps one live in peace.
- Bliss is the real attribute of the soul, while sorrow is an external element imposed on it.
- The highest state which a person can attain is to be identified with his ideal, where there is no sensation of attachment or aversion, no feeling of superiority or inferiority, and where there is a flow of consciousness. Problems and adverse conditions do not affect such people, for they have identified their goal.
- If a person is religious, he has a positive attitude towards every situation, and remains cheerful in every circumstance. This is difficult for an irreligious person.
- Practising meditation helps us to attain the ideal state.

3
THE INVISIBLE WORLD

One bright and sunny day, I came across a coconut tree. It had a trunk, long green leaves and bore fruit. That was all I could see but it was not everything that it had. There was much more to it—seeds, roots which I could not perceive.

Our senses cannot go beyond the visible, physical world. The invisible world is totally beyond our reach. The invisible, being inaccessible to our senses, can neither be affirmed nor fully denied. But it is not possible to understand the real meaning of life without understanding the invisible world. For it is the world where the secret of happiness lies.

EXISTENCE: THE COMBINED FORM OF THE VISIBLE AND THE INVISIBLE

Visibility and invisibility are relative concepts. Any variation in circumstance can make things visible or invisible. For instance, the coconut tree will no longer be visible if I move away from it. Even if there is a physical obstruction in front of it, the tree will no longer be seen.

The soul is invisible. Unlike the tree, the soul cannot be out of sight because man himself is a manifestation of the soul. He is a combination of the soul and the subtle invisible universe, which is made up of infinite atoms. Both the soul and the atoms are devoid of feelings like happiness, anger, sorrow. But the man who is at the meeting point of the two, that is, of the soul and the atoms, does experience such feelings. The pure soul is neither happy nor sad, neither bonded nor free. It is an experience of one's existence. When the soul is at the above-mentioned meeting point, it is susceptible to happiness, sadness, bondage and freedom. That is why attaining the purity of one's consciousness is treated as a state of freedom. That is the point where existence is at its zenith and where man overcomes all the constraints of his senses. He experiences absolute joy.

TYPES OF JOY

Joy is of two kinds:
- Momentary or materialistic joy
- Permanent or spiritual, absolute joy

Materialistic joy is easy, transient, interruptible and variable, and one which, normally, no one wants to abandon. In materialistic joy, the cycles of joy and sorrow go on. It is hard to calculate the number of times a man's mind varies between these two states in a single day. Hence, materialistic joy is also termed momentary joy. It is a subject of our direct perception.

Spiritual joy is difficult, invariable and uninterruptible. So, it is more reliable. In absolute or spiritual joy, a person remains forever in a state of joy, and the darkness of ignorance is absent.

Hence, it is also known as permanent joy. But it is difficult to understand because it is not a subject of our direct perception. If you want to live happily forever, you will have to understand its meaning and work for it.

Material pleasures are tangible because they are related to physical instruments. Only he who has felt a compelling attraction towards pure existence can abandon them. Spiritual joy is related to introspection. Once this complete knowledge has been acquired, the concept of joy undergoes a complete transformation. The complete light of knowledge is the first source of and the path to eternal happiness. Incomplete knowledge is the darkness in which a person is unable to find his way to his destination.

Complete knowledge includes knowledge of past, present and future. The man who has complete knowledge knows when to initiate the task and what its consequences will be. On the other hand, the man with incomplete knowledge does not have the understanding to initiate a task and is unaware of its consequences. So, he has to face misery at each and every step of his life.

An interesting story illustrates the above concept.

Once upon a time, there were two brothers. There was a vast difference in their financial conditions. The elder brother was rich whereas the younger brother did not have sufficient money even to buy his basic needs and to sustain his life. The elder brother never gave his younger brother a helping hand. Once, the younger brother, returning from the forest, saw an old man carrying wood. The old man asked, 'Why are you so sad?' The brother replied, 'I am hungry and there is nothing for me and my family to eat.' It was an angel disguised as an old man. He said, 'Do not worry. Carry this bundle of wood to my place and I'll give you something that will eliminate your sorrows.' The hungry brother did so. The old man rewarded him with a flour mill. The young man was surprised and said, 'What is the use of this flour mill to me? It would have been better if you had given me some money or food to eat.'

The old man replied: 'It is not an ordinary mill but a solution to your poverty and hunger. When you rotate it clockwise, it will give you whatever you desire. When you want to stop it, move it in the opposite direction.'

The man was overjoyed and, on reaching home, showed it to his wife. He narrated the story and the magic power of the flour mill. He asked her to make a wish and rotated the handle as instructed by the old man. To their surprise, there was a heap of rice in no time. Their joy and excitement knew no bounds. Gradually, they became rich and helped the poor and the needy of the town.

The elder brother grew jealous of his younger brother who had become rich almost overnight. He tried to find the reason behind his brother's sudden prosperity. As soon as he came to know about the magic flour mill and its effects, he decided to steal it.

Soon, he finalized his plan and announced that he was leaving town for a few days. He rented a boat and departed on his journey. On the way, while having lunch, he found that there was insufficient salt in his food. He thought of getting salt from the magic flour mill. He made his wish, moved the flour mill in a clockwise direction and the salt started pouring. It did not stop. The elder brother knew how to start the flour mill but not how to stop it. He regretted his mistake of not gaining complete knowledge. The small boat was drowned along with him.

This is the result of incomplete knowledge. It puts a man in a dangerous situation. One cannot think about eternal happiness in the absence of complete knowledge. The world is full of immorality, corruption, crime and violence which are increasing day by day. That is the result of delusion caused by incomplete knowledge.

PERCEIVING TRUTH THROUGH MEDITATION

Subtle truth can be perceived only by the subtle mind (psyche) and not by the gross mind. Practising 'preksha dhyana' helps train the subtle mind. The term 'preksha' means to see, to perceive. The mind has to be trained in the art of perception. Up to now, we have trained our minds in the art of thinking and so we are always busy thinking. Therefore, we have to impart fresh training to the mind so that it begins perceiving instead of thinking. Thinking takes place in the outer sphere of consciousness. Perception implies a deep penetration into the depths of consciousness. Once the mind has started perceiving, thinking subsides or becomes only a secondary occupation of the mind. In the absence of direct personal experience, we go on acquiescing uncritically to traditional ideas and views. We accept them as being true. The result is that, in critical situations, we are assailed by doubts and misgivings. Direct perception disperses doubts and misgivings, and gives us conviction. We often say, 'I have seen it with my own eyes.' What we mean is that, this is our perception. Perception is irrefutable proof of the existence of what has been perceived. Ordinarily, thinking comes first and perception occupies a secondary place. We have to reverse the order. First perceive, and then think.

For instance, in preksha meditation, we try to perceive the body. First, we see the form of the body, in its external appearance. Then we try to carry the mind into the body so that it may see the inner constituents of the body. We see the gross and the subtle vibrations of the body.

The human body is part and parcel of the universe in which we live. It is a replica of the universe. We try to perceive consciousness at all levels and to arouse and expand it. Perceiving the entire body means perceiving the cells and activating them. It is necessary to break the inertia of the cells so that they may become conscious. The conscious centres through which we perceive subtle things have to be freed from inertia. Meditative perception of the centres of consciousness is, therefore, to be repeated, over and over again. Ultimately, our super-sensuous consciousness becomes manifest and we can perceive the subtle truths.

ESSENCE

- It is not possible to understand the real meaning of life without understanding the invisible world.
- In materialistic joy, the cycle of joy and sorrow goes on.
- The complete light of knowledge is the first source of and the path to eternal happiness.
- Meditation is an important medium for attaining the light of complete knowledge.

4
KARMA: THE SEEDS OF JOY AND SORROW

When a person travels, he generally prefers to sit in the window seat to watch the picturesque view through the window. It is a general human tendency to get fascinated by the outer world. But the outer world is only a relative truth. The ultimate truth lies inside but most of us are indifferent to it. In Jain philosophy, the theory of karma is one of the fundamental theories. It is the basis to help us understand that the seeds of sorrow and joy—in fact, of every feeling, every circumstance we face—lie within us in the form of karma. Karma is one of the major reasons for sorrow. Some people are born in affluent and well-to-do families, while others have to battle against adverse conditions. This is not merely a philosophical discussion; we intend to describe the whole mechanism behind it.

The soul, by nature, is the same in each and every living organism. The pure form of the soul which we find in different organisms is the same, whether it is that of an elephant or an ant, of man or of God. The difference is due to the karma sharir attached to the soul. Karma sharir is formed and attached to the soul because of our deeds and acts. It is an imprint of our good, as well as bad, deeds.

A person can carry out three types of actions or deeds with his physical body:

- Mental
- Vocal
- Physical

All these actions, even the good ones, are accompanied by hidden malice—kashaya—and emotional impurities like anger, ego, dishonesty and greed. This leads to the bondage of karma with the soul. If the soul is totally free from kashaya, then there is no bondage of karma with the soul. Actions can be good as well as bad. Good actions lead to the accumulation of good karma, whereas evil actions result in bad karma.

One of the major elements that affect the bondage of karma is the intensity of the feelings attached to the act. The more intense the feeling, the more will be the karma. The more intense the karma, the more intense the feelings will be. A man who is always careful to keep his feelings and emotions pure will accumulate karma which is less intense and which he can shed more quickly. So, in order to be happy, one should lead a pious life, keeping one's feelings pure.

There is a well-known ancient story described in Jain philosophy. There lived a king named Prasannachandra who ruled over the small state of Potanpur. One day, he decided to renounce the world and entrusted his royal authority to his son.

Then Prasannachandra happened to come to Rajgriha with Lord Mahavira and started to meditate, standing on one leg.

Seeing his calm and quiet face, a minister of King Shrenik who was passing by, in a fit of jealousy and with the malicious intention of disturbing the monk's tranquillity, taunted him: 'Do you know what a terrible situation your son is in? You have become a carefree father, leaving your son, at a very young age, at the helm of affairs in your kingdom, which is surrounded by enemies. His life and the state are both at stake. If you have any feelings as a father, first save your child from danger. After that, you may think of spiritual attainment.'

Prasannachandra's mind grew restless though externally he was calm and unperturbed. He started visualizing his son's frightened face. He started a mental battle against the enemy. He wounded and killed all those who threatened his son's well-being. With mere feelings, he started accumulating intense karmas, karmas which were capable of taking him to the seventh hell—the lowest category of hell.

These agonizing states of mind, full of violence and fear, were contradictory to the peaceful nature that he was manifesting outwardly. New thoughts were continually fuelling the fire of wrath and vengeance burning within his mind. Suddenly, a humble man, seeing his external appearance, started to praise him: 'Leaving all the worldly pleasures and luxury and practising sadhana is indeed a noble deed.'

The monk quickly came to his senses: Whose son? Which empire? What am I thinking of? Why does this material world haunt me? What good can come of wishing harm to others? Such attachment is not wise. I must repudiate meaningless thoughts, such as those of victory and defeat. I wish to be beyond such trifles.

His thoughts were now redirected to their proper sphere. Prasannachandra had pure thoughts and a new vision. The mental war disappeared and the delusion was over. The veils of karma that had been obscuring knowledge and perception were flung aside and the path towards spiritual uplift was cleared. Prasannachandra obtained keval gyana and became omniscient.

The value of pure thinking can be clearly understood by this story. The purer the feelings and the thoughts, the less intense is the bondage of karmas. Impure feelings and thoughts result in a high-intensity bondage of karmas. Out of two persons engaged in the same activity, the one with detached feelings and less kashaya will have a smaller accumulation of karmas which can be shed easily, than the one who has intense feelings and more kashaya. The latter will have a bigger accumulation of karmas which are difficult to ward off and which remain for a longer time.

Thus, the soul is enclosed in a sheath of a contaminating field which produces radiation created by the karma sharir. The soul radiates psychic energy but the radiation has to pass through the karma sharir which contaminates it. During its passage, it interacts with kashaya and karma, forming a new field called the domain of adhyavasaya, that is, the primal psychic expression. It works in a systematic chain. The primal psychical expressions intermingle with the other subtle body, the tejas sharir. These compulsive forces, originating in the subtle body, first affect the endocrine system and compel it to secrete and distribute hormones that are responsible for mental, vocal and physical actions. Thus, the hormones become agents for executing the orders of primal drives in the physical body. Previous deeds act as a major hurdle, subordinating man's outlook, thinking, situations, behaviour and actions. This indirectly becomes the cause of sorrow.

The most interesting aspect of the karma theory is the transformation in the nature of karma, that is, the transformation of sorrow to happiness, and happiness to sorrow. A man's own actions, combined with psychic awareness, are the determining factors of his fate. Through his strong will power, he can think and act in such a way that it can transform the karma sharir. Here is an illustration explaining this aspect.

An astrologer once predicted the future of two brothers. He said that the older brother would be hanged within a few days while the younger one was destined to become a king. Both the brothers were taken aback by this forecast. The older brother thought that the astrologer's words might come true, it was better to be alert and cautious. With the fear of a violent death facing him, he altered his way of living through strenuous spiritual and moral efforts. The younger brother was quite pleased with the fact that he was soon going to be a king. He became extremely careless and reckless, and indulged in bad habits which degraded his karma. This began to empty the store of the good, pious karma that he had accumulated.

A few days later, the elder brother, while walking, was suddenly pricked by a thorn. The younger brother was passing through a jungle and he felt something hard beneath his foot. He dug the soil and found a pot filled with gold coins.

A few months passed by. Both the elder as well as the younger brother found that the astrologer's prediction in which they had seriously believed hadn't turned out to be true. They went to the astrologer and informed him that his prediction—about which he had been so sure—had not come true. The only major incident that had happened in the past few months was that the elder brother had been pricked by a thorn, and the younger brother had discovered a hidden pot filled with gold. The astrologer then asked the brothers about their behaviour during those months. After listening to them, the astrologer told the elder brother, 'You improved your behaviour and took up spiritual practices. So, you were only punished by a thorn.' He then turned to the younger brother and said, 'You were careless and, as a result of your bad deeds, your reward of a kingdom was turned into a small pot of gold.'

This proves that karma is the major driving force for joy and sorrow. Keeping this in mind, we should try to avoid committing bad deeds. Making mistakes, whether knowingly or unknowingly, is a common phenomenon. But we should always confess our guilt, which is a means of purifying one's self.

There are two concepts related to freeing the soul from karma. One is samvar and the other is nirjara. These concepts can be compared to a lake that is formed by a dam. Samvar is synonymous with closing the gates of the dam to prevent water from accumulating in the lake. In other words, it is the avoidance of actions which stop the accumulation of karma. Nirjara, on the other hand, is synonymous with opening the gates of the dam, and helping the outflow of the accumulated water. It is the act related to spiritual activities that are carried out by man for reducing and finally emptying the lake of karmas accumulated over countless births. One who is willing to be free of karmas should bring samvar and nirjara into practice. By practising these, one can attain eternal happiness and finally achieve moksha.

Thus, we should always keep in mind that we have to reform and rectify our mistakes, committed in the present as well as in past births. To lead a happy life, we should be vigilant over our present actions and alert about our future actions.

ESSENCE

- The theory of karma is one of the fundamentals of Jain philosophy.
- The soul, by its very nature, is the same in each and every organism.
- One of the major factors that affect the bondage of karma is the intensity of feelings attached to an act.
- The purer the feelings and thoughts, the less intense is the bondage of karma.
- The most interesting aspect of the karma theory is that its nature can be transformed.
- Samvara and nirjara are two steps for making oneself free from karmas.

MEDITATION: ANTARYATRA

1. POSTURE:
   Choose a posture in which you can sit comfortably and continually for forty-five minutes—full lotus, half lotus, cross-legged or diamond.

2. MUDRAS—THE POSITION OF THE HANDS (ANY ONE):
   i. Gyana Mudra:
      Place your right hand on the right knee and the left on the left knee, palms turned up. Touch the tip of the thumb to the tip of the index finger with a slight pressure. Keep the other fingers straight and relaxed.
   ii. Brahma Mudra:
      Place both hands on your lap, one above the other, palms turned up, the left palm under the right one. Keep your eyes softly closed.

3. RECITATION OF MAHAPRANA DHVANI:
   - Keep your lips softly closed, your spinal column and neck straight, without stiffness.
   - Inhale deeply and silently for about four to five seconds, with a calm mind, all muscles relaxed.
   - Concentrate on the top of your head.

- Keeping your lips together, exhale slowly, making the sound of mmm ……… through the nostrils, like the buzzing of a bee.
- This may last for eight to ten seconds. Inhale again and keep repeating this exercise for five minutes.

4. **KAYOTSARGA (RELAXATION):**
   - Relax all the muscles in your body.
   - Give an auto-suggestion to each and every muscle to relax and feel the muscles relaxing.
   - Release all the stress from your body.
   - Concentrate and allow your mind to travel, visiting all the parts of your body, from the big toe of your right foot to the top of the head.
   - Concentrate deeply and remain completely alert.

5. **ANTARYATRA (INTERNAL TRIP):**
   - Maintain the relaxed posture of the body, achieved by the process of total relaxation.
   - Focus your full attention on the bottom of the spine, the centre of energy. Direct it to travel upwards, along the spinal column to the top of the head, the centre of knowledge, and stay there for a moment. Then direct it to move downwards, taking the same path until you reach the centre of energy at the bottom of the spine. Repeat this exercise several times. Concentrate your entire attention on the path of the trip (the spinal

column) and do not permit it to be diverted.
- Carefully perceive the sensations caused by the subtle vibrations of the flow of the vital energy.
- After a little practice of this exercise, that is, the path of the ascending and descending mind, your attention must be synchronized with the rate of breathing. When the mind begins to ascend, start exhaling, so that the top of the head is reached simultaneously with the completion of the exhalation. Similarly, start the inhalation with the downward trip of the mind, and it should be completed when it reaches the centre of energy. Maintain the synchronization.

Conclude the meditation session by chanting the mahaprana dhvani three times.

5
DESIRE: THE ROOT CAUSE OF SORROW

According to *Acharangasutra*, a Jain scripture, if you want to get rid of sorrow you have to limit your desires. But it is very hard to move out from the world of desires. In this age of rapid economic development, when the world is moving towards materialism, the concept of limiting one's desires does not seem practical.

DESIRE: THE PATH FOR GROWTH OR SORROW?
Sorrow commences with the beginning of desire. According to economists, growth is directly proportional to wishes and desires. On the other hand, spiritualists believe that one's growth is inversely proportional to one's wishes and desires.

Economics is the discipline of material property while the science of peace rests on the limitation of wealth. There cannot be any meeting point between unlimited desires and peace. Does a man need only economic resources? If economic development is secured at the cost of peace, the ultimate result will be unhappy people who are unable to enjoy their economic prosperity. It is a basic requirement of the present times that there should be a combination of satisfaction of economic want and peace. A single-track approach will not solve the world's problems. Economics based on the satisfaction of wants and the economics of peace are complementary. Self-control, simplicity, giving up material comforts and limiting one's desires are not acceptable concepts to people who aspire to economic prosperity. Unlimited consumption, extravagance and material possessions are, no doubt, appealing. But there are also things that are not very tempting but are essential for the future of mankind.

Once, Acharyashree Tulsi was at Jain Vishva Bharati University, Ladnun (Rajasthan). Mrs Ahuja, vice chancellor of Kota University, visited him. During the conversation he said, 'Spirituality should be associated with economics in higher education.' Mrs Ahuja was surprised and said, 'How is that possible? Today's theory of economics says that an increase in desires will result in high growth, whereas spirituality asks us to restrain our desires in the interests of a peaceful life. How can they be reconciled?'

A relative viewpoint is the solution to this problem. It is true that life is hard with a total absence of desires but an excess of desires is harmful. A balance is required. Limited desires will not only result in development but also help us avoid unnecessary tension and stress.

WHY IS IT NECESSARY TO LIMIT DESIRES?
Today's young generation is attracted towards worldly pleasures. They want to accumulate more and more wealth. Their desires

are not limited to possessions; they want more fame, higher positions and unlimited power. On the contrary, if they want to lead a happy life, they must control their needs to a certain extent.

Wishes are never-ending. Everyone wants to fulfil all his desires in this one life, which is impossible to achieve. A student wants to get admission into college, but then he wants a good job. Once he gets a good job, he wants to grow and move up in the corporate hierarchy. His wishes keep on increasing. He keeps running to fulfil his desires but during this run, he forgets the true meaning of life.

Desires create stress which, in turn, affects and deteriorates one's mental and physical health. Today's generation is very aware of the credit card and its use. They use it thoughtlessly, going beyond their paying capacity, but at the time of paying their bills, many of them come under stress and tension. Here, an excess of desire creates unnecessary stress.

GREED VERSUS PEACE

Competition is a major reason for the increase in desire. A man, living comfortably in a bungalow, looks at his neighbour who has a higher standard of living and owns a multi-storeyed, state-of-the-art mansion, and becomes consumed by a desire to achieve the same, no matter how difficult it might be for him. He does not look at the one who is living in a small hut and who hardly gets two square meals a day, but has limited wants and is content. If he could see that, he would be satisfied and not unhappy. This makes it clear that an increase in wants and desire will lessen happiness, but a decrease in wants and desire will increase it.

CONTROLLED VERSUS UNCONTROLLED

There are two pictures of society before us:
- A society with uncontrolled desires, unlimited wants and uncontrolled consumption.
- A society with controlled desires, limited wants and restrained consumption.

A society in which desires are uncontrolled, where the needs are unlimited and where there is frivolous consumption, will be a sorrowful society. A society where desire, needs and consumption are under control will be a happy society.

In this world, everything is limited. The first principle of ecology is limitation. More consumers and a short supply; a limited supply and unlimited desires—how can these two be equated? Man has so many desires that they cannot all be fulfilled. Uncontrolled desires do not bring happiness to a person, they make him suffer.

The first cause of suffering and sorrow is boundless greed. It is never satisfied and, like an internal wound, it continually gives him pain. The second cause is want. Greed and want are camouflaged in the form of needs that go on multiplying, unsatisfied. The third cause is consumption. It is essential but ever since consumerism surfaced, it has expanded to an enormous extent, creating a huge impact on health, mind and consciousness.

Then there is the profile of another society—one with controlled desires, controlled wants and controlled consumption. A man who controls his wants will never become unhappy. He is aware that he cannot fulfil all his wishes. As a corollary, he limits his wants, shutting the door on unhappiness.

The basic needs of life do not bother a man but unrealistic wants harass him. The wants which trouble him are those which are generated artificially by imaginary needs. These wants create a disposition towards consumption. Eventually, temptation takes a dominant position and the real needs lose their meaning.

CLASSIFICATION ACCORDING TO DESIRE
Lord Mahavira classified man into three categories:
- One with many desires (mahechha)
- One with a few desires (alpechha)
- One with no desires (anichha)

MAHECHHA
Today's economy wants us to multiply our desires. If there is an increase in wants then there is inspiration for initiative, leading to greater efforts. When there are few wants there are few efforts. Mahavira, while analysing both the characteristics, said that the one who has great desires has many wants. He might earn his living by immoral means. He might become violent, furious, or wicked, and he will not have consideration for anybody or anything. If it is in his self-interest, he might not even hesitate to kill somebody.

Today, innocent, dumb animals and birds are being killed thoughtlessly for manufacturing luxury products and cosmetics. This is being done merely for the sake of money. Large amounts of money cannot be earned without violence, cheating, manipulation and fraud.

It is imperative that we think of the welfare of others, along with what is right. Without controlling our wants and limiting our desires, we cannot carry out welfare.

ALPECHHA
A man with alpechha does have desires, but they are limited. Such a person, for instance, will set up a factory but he will

not accumulate too much wealth for himself. The policy of decentralized economy and decentralized power about which Mahatma Gandhi talked is the reiteration of what Mahavira called few desires and few wants. Mahavira said, 'Dhammenag vitte kappemana' (a person with few wants earns his living virtuously).

The basic difference between a person with alpechha and one with mahechha is one of ethics and moral values. I would like to mention here the example of Shrimad Rajchandra, who gave the basic mantra of ahimsa to Mahatma Gandhi. Shrimad Rajchandra entered into a deal with a jewellery trader. All of a sudden, the prices shot up. The trader started losing fifty thousand rupees in just a single consignment. Shrimad Rajchandra called upon the trader and asked him to take out the agreement. The trader said, 'Sir, you need not worry. I will pay you the entire amount. But, at present, I am not in a position to do so.' Shrimad Rajchandra replied, 'I am not talking about the payment. I just want to see that agreement once.'

The trader thought that, after getting back the agreement, Rajchandra would file a case in court and he would be trapped. So he was reluctant to give the agreement but eventually there was no way out. On receiving the agreement, Shrimad Rajchandra tore it into pieces and assured the trader, 'Rajchandra can drink poison but he cannot suck anybody's blood. I am cancelling the deal.'

Such a humane act can only be performed by a person who has compassion in his heart. He cannot be unjust, he does not behave ruthlessly, nor does he exploit others. He does not manipulate nor does he try to take away someone else's possessions.

ANICHHA

The third category of person is the one who has controlled his wants.

Once, Lord Buddha was visiting Pataliputra. Several people approached him with their problems. He preached them, listened to them and solved their problems. One day, after his sermon, at which many dignitaries, including the king, were present, Anand, the disciple of Buddha, asked, 'What is joy? Who is the happiest person in this assembly?'

Buddha was silent for a few minutes and looked around. There was pin-drop silence and everyone was eager to hear the answer. People thought that it would be the king or the rich people present there. But surprisingly, Lord Buddha pointed to a lean and thin poor man.

The people were confused by his answer. Understanding their confusion, Buddha asked everyone to list their needs. Everyone, except the man to whom Buddha had pointed, presented their long list of desires to him.

At last Buddha questioned the poor man, 'What do you need?' The man replied, 'Nothing. But since you have asked, I would like to be free of all kinds of needs.' Anand asked, 'Don't you want money, new clothes, anything else?' The poor man replied, 'No. I am happy.' The people assembled there had received their answer.

Such a person has conquered his desires. He often becomes detached from society by becoming a saint. He does not carry out any economic activities. His life is devoted to sadhana. Though, in this era, there are very few such people, during Lord Mahavira's time, there was no dearth of them. When Swami Vivekananda travelled to Europe and the US, the people there were astonished by his lifestyle. They wondered how anyone could live such a restricted life, free of material desires.

It is impossible for everyone to lead a life totally devoid of desires. But, to have a happy and peaceful life, we must try to restrain ourselves from entertaining unnecessary desires. This will not only make our lives better but also this earth a better place to live in.

ESSENCE

- Desire is the origin of sorrow. To avoid sorrow, one must limit one's desires.
- Today, economists believe in the necessity of desires for achieving growth, whereas spiritualists believe in restraining them for one's personal growth. The relative viewpoint is that limited desires come as a solution here.
- Excessive desires create stress and tension, give rise to unnecessary competition and greed, and disturb mental peace.
- Boundless greed, unnecessary wants and excess consumption result in sorrow.
- A society with controlled desires will be happy, whereas one with unlimited needs will be sorrowful.
- A man on the basis of his desires can be classified as:
  - One with many desires (mahechha)
  - One with a few desires (alpechha)
  - One with no desires (anichha)

6
ANGER: THE FIRE THAT BURNS HAPPINESS

Anger is one of the biggest problems of the present age. Every day the newspapers are filled with incidents of domestic violence and hostility among the youths. The major cause of it is uncontrolled anger.

There are various reasons for it. According to medical science, the hypersecretion of adrenal glands triggers the emotions of man. Psychologists say that the instinct for fighting causes anger. Ayurveda believes that an imbalance of bile makes a man angry. According to Jain philosophy, the rise of mohaniya karma (deluding karma) is the hidden cause of anger.

Anger is a fundamental instinct of the human being. Everybody knows that anger is not good, and yet, people cannot prevent themselves from getting angry. There are various factors that lead to anger, like ego, possessiveness and unfulfilled desires. It is not limited to age. A child asks for something which a mother may refuse. The child gets angry and cries. When the child becomes uncontrollable, the mother reacts and becomes angry. A serious problem that the world faces today is anger that arises for no apparent reason. It is anger which gets accumulated within and makes the modern man anxious and agitated.

The primary reason for unreasoning or blind anger is that man, right from his childhood, is exposed to the external world without any imprint of spirituality on him. Second, there is often a lack of empathetic company with whom he can share his feelings; this leads to a feeling of suffocation caused by accumulated emotions. Third, the ego is nourished from a very young age.

ANGER IS OF TWO FORMS:
- Saphalikaran
- Viphalikaran

If, on getting angry, a person utters abusive words, fights or becomes physically violent, then such behaviour is known as saphalikaran.

If a man does not react physically or use abusive words and keeps himself calm even when he is angry, then such behaviour is known as viphalikaran.

ANGER IS OF TWO TYPES:
One is like a line drawn in the sand, which disappears when the wind blows. A man of this type becomes normal within a few seconds after getting angry.

The second is like a line engraved in stone, which will not disappear even if a thunderbolt strikes, and which will remain there for a very long time. A man of this type finds it difficult to get back to his normal self after getting angry.

Often, people who work in the administrative sector knowingly display their anger. According to them, if they don't get angry with people working under them, they will not be taken seriously. I think this is a misconception among many people. If they try to explain in a polite manner, the workers will understand and carry out the orders. On the other hand, if the boss explains the same thing in an angry tone, the workers will understand that the job has to be done but will harbour a feeling of resentment towards the boss.

Once, a corporal was carrying out orders to load some cargo. He was shouting at the workers who were trying hard to lift the load. A man who was passing by saw this, went up to the corporal and asked what the problem was. The corporal told him that they needed one more worker to complete the work. The passer-by said, 'Why don't you help them?' The corporal, proud of his status, replied arrogantly, 'How can a man of my rank do such an inferior job? These workers are of no use. If you are so concerned, why don't you help them?' The man readily helped the workers, and the cargo was loaded successfully. When the corporal later inquired who the man was, he felt ashamed. The man was George Washington, who was a high-ranking officer then and later became the first president of the United States. The incident shows that a humble and polite manner is the best way of getting your orders carried out. One can earn respect only through it and not through anger.

DISADVANTAGES OF ANGER:

- ☞ Some people, on getting angry, use harsh words which hurt others deeply. This gives rise to negative feelings and increases conflicts within families and with friends. **When a person becomes angry, he gets out of control.**

For instance, a husband screamed at his wife and asked her to go away thinking he didn't need her any more. A few days later, he regretted his behaviour and realized his need for his wife. History is full of examples where an angry king expels his minister but needs him later to help him run his country smoothly. The king feels ashamed of his behaviour and recalls his old minister after undergoing a lot of troubles.

- Anger reduces vital energy. It is said that one spurt of anger consumes nine hours of a body's vital energy. So, those who lose their temper frequently should ponder the amount of vital energy they lose every day.
- Anger affects even physical health. When people get angry, their body shakes, lips vibrate and eyes become blood red. Anger also disturbs the different systems of the body. It weakens the digestive system and has a bad effect on the circulatory system.
- A group of villagers visited me. They introduced themselves but I couldn't find one member of their family whom I had known well. So I inquired after him. They replied, 'He passed away.' I asked, 'How can it be possible! He was so healthy and showed no signs of any major disease.' They said, 'One day, he lost his temper and screamed at his servant. At that very minute, he got a severe heart attack and died.' Anger is thus a terrible disease which can even take lives.
- Anger reduces our mental strength. It badly affects the human mind, reducing memory power, imagination and the ability to think. This is why people who get angry respond slowly. Anger is a major obstacle especially in the development of children. Those

children who frequently throw tantrums do not have a sharp memory. Such children are often not able to score good marks, and could even end up taking harsh steps like committing suicide, thereby creating trouble for their families. Since anger influences imagination and thinking power, a man who often loses his temper cannot contribute significantly to his own development and the society's.

- Anger makes our wavelengths negative, affecting others too.
- Once, a woman from Mumbai visited me. She was short-tempered and wanted a solution for her anger. I suggested that she practise preksha dhyana. After a few days, she visited me again. This time she had a new question. She said, 'My husband is fond of eating a variety of dishes. So, I used to cook different kinds of food for him but he always found fault in them. However, nowadays, he says, "You have magic in your fingers, whatever you cook tastes sweet." Why is that? I want to know the reason for this change.' I told her, 'It is very simple. You were short-tempered before. While cooking, you used to add your anger to the food, which made it taste bitter. But now you add forgiveness which makes the food sweet.'

Now the question arises, how can one gain control over one's anger? There are certain methods by which this can be done.

EXPERIMENTS FOR CONTROLLING ANGER:

- It would be easy to endure all kinds of situations—favourable and adverse—if we practised long and rhythmic breathing. In a state of excitement, one cannot tolerate anything. By practising long breathing we can be greatly benefited. In an adverse situation, when the mind flares up with excitement, immediately start taking long breaths. You will feel as if a barrier has intervened between fire and water.

Water is wasted when it is used to extinguish fire. But if water is filled in a pot and is placed on the fire, it gets heated up and becomes a thing of utility. The process of breathing may be compared to such a pot. If this pot of water is put to the right use, the fire becomes a useful tool and whatever it achieves is not wasted. The energy used here is saved and becomes a productive power.

- If we want to control anger we should concentrate on the frontal lobe which is the field of emotion. In preksha dhyana, it is known as the centre of peace, the centre of enlightenment. It is here that the fire of tolerance burns. The emotional area of the brain is also the seat of excitement and intolerance. Without controlling it, the capacity for tolerance cannot be developed. An effective method of transforming the emotional area is to concentrate on the centre of enlightenment and the centre of peace. These are two practical exercises which can help control and pacify the area of emotional pain. The greater the control, the less the excitement.
- If we want to avoid anger, we must do some research into why it is bad. Why do we want to avoid it? If there were nothing wrong with it, the question of refraining from it would not rise. Is anger bad? We must reflect upon it. We must dissect it, practise anupreksha, go deep

into it, and reach a state of perceptual judgement and reflective analysis.

Then only will we come to know that anger is a kind of fever. When it enters the body it invades it and impairs one's powers. It is a fever of the brain, of the heart and of the adrenal glands. It saps the vitality from all three. When a man gives way to anger, it is the brain that gets affected, first and foremost. It gets totally flushed. There is a terrible expense of energy because of perturbation, and each and every part of the brain becomes burning hot. The heart is the second victim of anger. The moment a man is overcome by anger, the heartbeats register a sudden increase. The heart palpitates faster and starts functioning erratically. The adrenal glands are the third victims of wrath. While a man is in a state of rage, they are obliged to secrete more and more, and their potency gets diminished. Because of anger, the brain, the heart and the adrenal glands are all severely affected, and the vitality of all three is undermined. These three constitute important elements of life. The slightest retardation of the brain upsets the entire nervous system. With the weakness of the heart, the circulatory system goes out of order. And a malfunctioning of the adrenal glands can have serious consequences on one's health.

These are the consequences of anger. This is an analysis of its effects. When, in the course of practising contemplation, we reach this stage, we understand that anger must not only be controlled, it must be avoided.

Then the question arises: is it possible for us to avoid anger? The spiritual practitioner ruminates upon it, and he discovers that he has in him an unlimited capacity for avoiding it. Having realized this fact, he reaches the next stage of contemplation—

discretion. The spiritual practitioner says to himself, 'I can renounce anger because anger is not me. Anger is not my nature. Had anger been my nature, I could have never renounced it. No man can get away from his real nature. But I am not anger. I am different from anger. I am knowledge. I am bliss. Anger only clouds my knowledge; it distorts my vision and vitiates my bliss. It destroys my power.' Contemplating thus, he realizes that he is not anger and anger is not his nature.

ESSENCE

- Anger is the biggest problem of the present times that man, irrespective of his age, faces.
- Anger is of two forms—saphalikaran, where a person becomes violent, and viphalikaran, where a person keeps calm.
- Anger can be classified as being of two types—one which disappears in a few seconds, and another that lingers for a longer time.
- Disadvantages of anger:
    - Creates conflicts within families and with friends;
    - Reduces vital energy;
    - Affects physical health;
    - Reduces mental strength;
    - Makes our wavelengths negative, thereby affecting others.
- Experiments in controlling anger:
    - Long, slow breathing;
    - Concentrating on the emotional area, that is, the centre of peace and the centre of enlightenment;
    - Practising anupreksha, that is, self-analysis.
- The three major victims of anger are the brain, the heart and the adrenal glands.
- Contemplating on 'I am not anger and anger is not my nature' helps the spiritual practitioner realize the unlimited capacity he has to renounce anger.

7
CAN SORROW BE REDUCED?

It has been accepted from ancient times that meditation can reduce the effects of sorrow. But today's generation is constantly bothered about its relevance in modern times. To examine its truth, we must first understand the cause of sorrow.

There are various causes of sorrow. The major causes can be divided into four categories:

1. IMAGINATION
Human development is the result of a wonderful brain with imagination as one of its major functions. But this imagination can turn out to be either a boon or a bane.

Imagination can be categorized as:
- Positive imagination
- Negative imagination

Imagination which is based on realistic parameters—like setting goals, planning, visualizing a positive future—is an example of a positive imagination. Such an imagination is desirable and becomes a stepping stone to a bright future. On the other hand, the unwanted imagination born out of negative emotions, like fear, jealousy, greed or hatred, is a negative imagination. A man creates his own world of sorrow by falling prey to such imagination that has no basis in reality.

An example: A wise man was called in to advise a couple who were quarrelling over the future of their child. The mother said, 'I am in poor health and have to visit the doctor very often. In fact, half the household budget goes on my medical expenses. It would be wonderful if our child was trained as a doctor. My treatment costs would come to an end then.'

The father thought differently. 'I spend a lot of time and money on various cases filed in the court', he said. 'And the lawyers charge me heavily for their expertise. If our child became a lawyer it would save me both time and money.'

The wise man said that he understood both points of view but wanted to meet the child so he could get the child's opinion on the matter. At that point, the quarrelling couple confessed that the child had not yet been born.

Such imaginative thoughts can create a web of sorrow for us. Now the question is, 'Can meditation provide the solution to such problems?' This illusionary imagination is the result of the fickleness of our mind and over-thinking. Meditation guides us to a state where we can go beyond our thoughts, where there is no sign of imaginary sorrow.

2. SCARCITY

A lack of resources, an absence of livelihood and a scarcity of the primary necessities can lead to a sorrowful condition. Now, how can meditation remove sorrow caused by scarcity? It seems impossible to prove that meditation can free a person from sorrow created by poverty, but a deeper insight will definitely give a ray of hope.

Hiuen Tsang, a renowned Chinese philosopher of his time, was once visited by a rich merchant named Sikung. In order to reach the philosopher's abode, the merchant had to leave his carriage and walk through increasingly narrow lanes in a poor neighbourhood. He reached a shabby hut. Hiuen Tsang came to welcome him, wearing his old, much-mended garments and a cap made of leaves.

Sikung was shocked by the philosopher's condition and said, 'You seem to be very poor and leading a miserable life.'

Hiuen Tsang answered. 'Sikung, I am poor but not sorrowful. People who are ignorant become unhappy and moan about their condition. I am neither ignorant nor sorrowful.'

There is a clearly drawn line dividing poverty and sorrow. It is lack of knowledge that gives rise to sorrow. An ignorant person stumbles at every step due to his false notions. In fact, people with minimum resources often lead happy lives whereas the rich may lead stressful and sorrowful lives.

Since ancient times, in Indian culture, there has been a tradition of renunciation. Many, including emperors, have chosen this path and achieved eternal bliss. If scarcity had been the real cause of sorrow, then sages and holy men too, who renounce their worldly possessions and depend on alms for basic necessities, would have been sorrowful. But they have led happy and satisfied lives, secure in their possession of knowledge.

Ignorance, rather than scarcity, is the real cause of sorrow. Scarcity can create poverty but not sorrow. Only scarcity combined with ignorance gives rise to sorrow. If scarcity had been the cause of sorrow, then the tradition of renunciation would have been erroneous. This actually proves that the real cause of sorrow is ignorance and not scarcity.

The light attained through meditation can dispel the darkness of ignorance. When the lamp of awareness is lit, the difference between scarcity and sorrow becomes clear. This will alter our outlook and remove the perception that scarcity leads to distress.

3. SEPARATION

The world is a cycle of union and separation. Love and affection create a bond between parents and children, between husband and wife, between close friends. But it is a law of nature that no union is permanent. The law of birth and death signifies union and separation.

Once, a lady who had lost her husband four years earlier participated in a preksha meditation camp. She was quite distressed and expressed her feelings, saying, 'I am trying to overcome the grief over my husband's demise, but I cannot. The thought of being separated from him keeps haunting me. Sometimes I feel it would be better for me to die.'

Her sorrow seemed to be unending. I thought at that moment what could be the remedy for this sorrow. Could meditation prove to be the solution here? But when we try to analyse, we realize that it is not the parting which is the root cause of sorrow but the false notion which we attach to separation. We refuse to accept the fact that separation is inevitable.

There is an impressive story about Ravi Meher, a school teacher, who used to say, 'God has given us this life and even if he takes it back, what is there to be upset about? We should be thankful for the time he has granted us.'

CAN SORROW BE REDUCED?

He had a wife and two children whom he loved dearly. An epidemic struck his village one summer and very swiftly claimed the lives of his two children. When he came home from work and called for his children, his wife took him to the room where their children were laid out, wrapped in white sheets. Meher was shocked and grief-stricken but his wife reminded him, 'You have always said that our lives were a gift from God and that he could take back his gift whenever he desired.' Meher recognized the truth and calmed down. Accepting the universal truth, he set out to perform the last rites.

If we assume separation to be the cause of sorrow then it should make everyone sad and miserable. The Meher couple had to face separation but they accepted it with equanimity. It seems to be an extraordinary task but it is not impossible. Separation leads one to false notions which fills one with sorrow. In the absence of these false notions, separation may occur but will not be accompanied by sorrow. Sorrow is not the obvious concomitant of scarcity or separation.

Many people are afraid of death. Here, the issue is not separation from another person; it is separation from life itself. They crave eternal life. Such men live lives full of sorrow. People who acknowledge the universal truth of separation are free from the fear of death. They lead a stress-free life.

Various religions and philosophies preach the art of living but in the Jain tradition, the art of dying is also taught. A person gets the opportunity to live for many years but there is only one single chance of dying. The duration of life is long but death occurs in a single moment. A man may live a miserable long life, but then, why should he be scared of death?

Familiarity with the art of dying eases the burden of death and turns the painful moment into a celebration. The technique alters the mental state of a person. Now death is no longer threatening. The mind is prepared to welcome death and to celebrate it as a joyous occasion.

In the Jain tradition, there is a concept of a lifelong fast, a procedure to prepare oneself for death. The duration is of twelve years. When a person feels that he has crossed a certain age and that his senses are becoming feeble and that he is becoming dependent on others, he moves from worldly affairs to spiritual ones; he practises penance, meditation, reads religious literature and awakens his spiritual self. The technique of spiritual death negates the sorrow emanating from the separation of the soul and the body.

4. ENVIRONMENT AND SURROUNDINGS

Everyone wants to live happily and comfortably but as soon as adversity enters our lives we tend to become sorrowful. Adversity and sorrow appear to be synonymous. Is there an intimate relationship between sorrow and adversity? The answer is no. We are all bound to meet with adversity at some point of time but it is up to us how we meet it and how we react to it. It is our attitude towards adversity that determines our joy and our sorrow.

Pleasure and adversities, both depend on our assumptions. We form our own notions that some things are more favourable and others are less favourable or desirable. Our own reactions and thoughts on what we conceive to be unfavourable create more sorrow. Through meditation, these emotions can be controlled and a person can remain calm and peaceful in any condition.

A guru and his disciple were sitting together. A stranger came up and started abusing them. Both listened for a while, but after some time the disciple was filled with anger and could not control himself. He started shouting at the stranger. At that, the guru immediately left the place. The disciple, baffled by his guru's behaviour, asked him, 'All this while, you were calmly listening to the man's insults, but when I retaliated, why did you desert me?' The guru replied, 'Until now, a devil was standing before me and I was sitting with a divine soul. But then there were two devils in front of me, so, it seemed better to leave the place.'

We should understand clearly that sorrow is a by-product of our outlook on life. The main cause of sorrow is the materialistic outlook. A spiritual outlook frees one from sorrow that is caused by a negative imagination, and ignorance that is caused by scarcity, separation and adversity. Hence, changing one's outlook from materialistic to spiritual, developing a new attitude and accepting the universal truths can liberate one from sorrow.

MEDITATION: A SOLUTION

The practical approach to dealing with sorrow is antaryatra, the inner journey, a technique of preksha meditation. By practising it, one can achieve a spiritual outlook that negates sorrow. During the inner journey, one travels between the psychic centres of the body—from the centre of energy located at the base of the spinal cord to the centre of knowledge located at the crown of the skull. These two centres act like two end poles. When the flow of vital energy travels from the lower to the upper pole, it brings our consciousness from outside to inside. Our attention moves from the outer senses to an inner spiritual awakening. This process, in conjunction with proper breathing, is a source of tremendous energy. It can help us transform our nature and thinking patterns. It can open the door to eternal peace and happiness.

ESSENCE

- There are four major causes of sorrow: imagination, scarcity, separation, and environment and surroundings.
- A negative imagination creates a web of sorrow that has no existence in reality.
- Not scarcity alone, but scarcity accompanied by ignorance, is the real cause for sorrow.
- Sorrow is not the obvious concomitant of scarcity or separation. Separation leads us to false notions which make us suffer.
- Familiarity with the art of dying—a technique for a spiritual death—eases the burden of death and negates the sorrow emanating from the separation of the soul and the body.
- Our attitude towards adversity determines our joy and sorrow. Sorrow emanates when we conceive things to be unfavourable.
- Sorrow is a by-product of our outlook on life. Developing a spiritual instead of a materialistic outlook, cultivating a new attitude, and accepting the universal truths free one from all causes of sorrow.

8
STRESS AND SORROW

Joy and sorrow are the two words on the basis of which a man's personality can be analysed. They depend on a man's actions, thought processes and his inclinations. To make this clearer, one should know that there are four types of sorrow: physical sorrow, mental sorrow, emotional sorrow and karmic sorrow.

Physical sorrow is so interconnected with the other three that it cannot be fully defined without referring to them. It makes up the largest part of the sorrow that we feel in day-to-day life. In today's world of technology, industrialization and urbanization, we are constantly subjected to tremendous stress and tension. The biggest problem that man faces today is that he is continually over-pressurized, he is always restless, and this leads to stress. Modern man has become a 'patient of the mind'. This has resulted in a rise in the number of people who, at a very young age, suffer from hypertension, heart ailments and high blood pressure.

Ancient medicine classifies diseases into two types: those caused by external agents and those produced by internal agents. According to Ayurveda, the imbalance of internal agents, like vata (air), pitta (bile) and kapha (phlegm), stimulate disease. According to naturopathy, the accumulation of toxins in our system makes us unhealthy. According to Jain philosophy, karma—the imprint of deeds done in the previous birth—becomes the cause of pain and illness.

STRESS AND ITS MECHANISM

Man's life, set to an incredibly fast pace, has become a mere rat race. He keeps running after one thing or the other. Quick and fast actions create a stressful condition.

Any condition that needs behavioural adjustments is termed as a stressful condition. Dr Hans Selye, an international authority on stress, defines stress as 'the rate of wear and tear of the body'. He shows that cold, heat, rage, drugs, excitement, pain, grief and even joy activate the stress mechanism in the same way. If the stress is physical—such as excessive cold—the skin density and the breathing change, the blood vessels at the surface contract. Whenever one encounters a psychologically stressful situation, an elaborate innate mechanism is automatically put into action. This mechanism involves:

- Hypothalamus—the remarkable part of the brain which integrates all the functions of the body which are not normally controlled by the conscious mind.
- Pituitary gland—called the master of the endocrine system because it regulates other glands.
- Adrenal gland—which secretes adrenalin and other hormones to keep the body tense and alert.
- The sympathetic component of the autonomic nervous

system whose responsibility is ultimately to prepare the body for the 'fight-or-flight' response.

The psychological conditions which are brought about by the integrated action of the above are:

- The blood supply to the digestive system is curtailed; digestion is slowed down or halted.
- The salivary glands dry up.
- The respiration rate increases, the breathing becomes faster or comes in gasps.
- The liver releases some of the store of blood sugar which is carried to the muscles of the arms and the legs.
- The heart beats faster to pump more blood where it is most needed, and the blood pressure rises.

All these and many other complex changes occur to generate extra quantities of the electrochemical and hormonal energy which enable us to act quickly. The energy goes to the muscles even when there is nothing that needs to be done, and energy bounds up in the muscles as tension. When the emergency conditions have subsided, we have what is needed to bring us back to a balanced, tensionless state. It is the concern of the other component of the autonomic nervous system—the parasympathetic—to resume normal activity and restore peaceful conditions. The parasympathetic nervous system is designed to work in close harmony and balance with the sympathetic nervous system. The activation of the parasympathetic is meant to happen naturally after the emergency is over. Its response is to balance the sympathetic by returning the biochemistry to normal and by relaxing the tense muscles. The sympathetic nervous system is action-oriented and aggressive; the parasympathetic nervous system is restorative and passive. When both function normally, there is a see-saw action which reflects in our body as rhythmic cycles of action and rest. When the equilibrium breaks down, there is a dangerous tension. Since modern lifestyles always keep us on the go, the restoring apparatus—the parasympathetic nervous system—seldom gets a chance to operate fully. That is, our muscles and nerves hardly ever return to their natural condition.

DISORDERS CAUSED BY STRESS OR TENSION

All animals, including human beings, possess this innate mechanism, and its response which prepares one for fight or flight is involuntary. If a stressful situation recurs regularly, the stress mechanism gets repeatedly activated. If the psychological conditions described above persist over a long time or recur frequently, serious disorders can occur. Thus, if the blood pressure remains high and the blood vessels get constricted, the result will be a heart attack or a stroke; if the reduced blood supply to the stomach is prolonged, there will be digestive disorders; if the breathing continues at a high rate, it may result in asthma. Sustained muscle tension will cause aches and pains in the head, back, neck and shoulders. Besides this, the chronic tension may also bring on feelings of panic and irrational fear which could be frightening, even crippling. The modern man, tense, nervous and anxious, is driven inexorably into stress because his constant state of anxiety prevents him from coping with the relentless demands of today's life. There is plenty of evidence now to show that tension may play a significant part in promoting or triggering a great many illnesses. If we want to successfully solve the problems of stress, we have to find a way of allowing the parasympathetic nervous system to function efficiently, so that it can re-establish the equilibrium and harmony which has been destroyed.

CURE IS ALSO INHERENT

Modern lifestyles are most unlikely to change for the better. Sure, we have developed pharmaceutical wonder drugs in the form of tranquillizers, which give temporary relief. In the long run, however, the medicine itself creates more serious problems than the original disease. The question is: Are we then destined to be doomed by our environmental conditions or are we capable of adapting ourselves so as to avoid, at least, the more injurious effects of daily stress?

Fortunately, we also possess an inner mechanism which produces physiological conditions, which are diametrically opposite to the fight-or-flight response. Swiss physiologist Walter Rudolph Hess, winner of the 1949 Nobel Prize in Physiology, described its response as a protective mechanism against overstress, promoting restorative processes, and called it a 'trophotropic response'. Herbert Benson, M.D., has termed this reaction 'relaxation response'.

It is possible to train ourselves to activate the protective mechanism and to influence our reactions to stress. The increased secretion and output of adrenaline can be normalized and the sympathetic dominance counter-balanced by an increased parasympathetic activity. Regular practice of kayotsarga is a potent remedy for the dangerous diseases of modern times.

RELAXATION

Kayotsarga is a form of relaxation which is a direct and harmless way of relaxing tension. One cannot hope to enjoy either health or happiness so long as one is under the insidious influence of tension in spite of possessing the amenities and luxuries of life. Anybody who, after learning the technique, practises systematic relaxation for thirty to forty-five minutes, will remain relaxed and unperturbed in any situation.

When we sleep, our nerves and muscles are in a relaxed position. When we rest, there is a weak nerve impulse and the muscles are in a quiescent state. When we move or are engaged in some physical activity, the nerve impulse increases and the muscles contract. All the three states described above normally occur many times a day. The fourth state—abnormal yet frequent—is the state of hypertension. Perpetually tightened jaws, clenched teeth, frowning brows and hardened abdominal muscles are some of the visible signs of this state. In this state, a strong nerve impulse is generated, leaving the muscles in an unnecessary permanent contraction.

With conscious and voluntary actions, it is possible to switch off this impulse to the muscles which is more efficient than sleep. Sleep is seldom refreshing. In kayotsarga, the flow of impulse is reduced to nil and the output of energy to the minimum. It is so effective that it can relieve tension and fatigue more effectively in half an hour than many hours of indifferent sleep can. However, it cannot be achieved by force, constraint or violence. It is an exercise of the mastery of the conscious will over the body by the technique of auto-suggestion. With its help, one can remain relaxed under the most exasperating conditions. Kayotsarga is a form of faith healing where the patient himself controls the process, relaxing each body part in turn by coaxing auto-suggestion.

Kayotsarga helps counteract the sympathetic dominance. This alleviates other emotional aspects, like mitigating various anxiety states and treating some cardiac problems. A cessation of the unnecessary voluntary movements of body and speech brings about discipline in the sense organs.

According to Jain philosophy, the gross physical body is the medium for the perception of suffering or its manifestation but not its root cause. The root cause is the most subtle body called karma sharir—the coded record of one's past deeds. It is responsible for motion, agitation and tension caused in daily life. Kayotsarga is actually a process for searching and finding the root of all miseries and sufferings. In the state of kayotsarga, one is able to detect and identify the root cause of mundane suffering. And once this truth is known, there is a fundamental change in the attitude towards the gross body. Kayotsarga is the first war against the enemy—karma sharir. It helps one reach the state of self-awareness, where the journey to self-realization commences.

KAYOTSARGA: RELAXATION

For a successful session of meditation practice, it is necessary to relax the whole body and to eliminate muscular tension. Relaxation and meditation are not identical, but the latter cannot be performed properly unless the body becomes motionless. As long as the body is tense and the muscles contracted, the free flow of energy (prana) is inhibited and mental steadiness and concentration are not possible. Kayotsarga is thus an essential pre-condition of meditation practice.

Kayotsarga is not only total relaxation of the body but also a real experience of self-awareness.

1. POSTURE:

Normally, relaxation is to be done in a lying-down position, but it can also be done in a sitting posture. Before lying down, create a suitable atmosphere for the exercise. Standing up, recite loudly, 'It is essential for me to relax to get rid of the physical, mental and emotional tensions. I shall devote myself wholly to the exercise of relaxation.' Having resolved thus, try to set aside your worries. Standing on your toes, take a deep breath, and stretch out fully, extending your arms above your head. Repeat this three to four times. Then

KAYOTSARGA: RELAXATION

lie down and repeat the stretching operation another three to four times.

2. INSTRUCTIONS:
- Maintain the posture, keeping the spine and neck straight but without stiffness, eyes softly closed. Relax all the muscles of your body and let them become limp.
- Concentrate your mind on each part of the body, one by one. Allow each part to relax by the process of auto-suggestion and feel that it has relaxed.
- Starting with the big toe of the right foot, allow your mind to spread throughout the toe, suggesting to the muscles and the nerves that they relax; experience the resulting relaxation and pass on to the other parts of the right leg—the other toes, sole, heel, ankle, upper part of the foot, calf muscles, knee, thigh and buttock. In the same way, relax the left limb up to the hip joint.
- Next, relax the trunk from the hip joint to the neck, starting with the back and the front of the lower and the upper abdomen, going up to the ribs—front and back, the chest muscles, the collar bone up to the neck muscles. Then relax both limbs from palms to the shoulders, that is, the right hand—thumb, fingers, palm,

UNDERSTANDING JOY AND SORROW

wrist, lower arm, elbow, upper arm and shoulder. Similarly, the left hand.
- Finally, relax the head from the neck to the throat, chin, jaws, lips, mouth, cheeks and all the other facial muscles, nose, eyes, ears, temples, forehead and scalp.
- Experience the relaxed state of the whole body. Retain the relaxed condition throughout the meditation session.

Conclude the meditation session by chanting the mahaprana dhvani three times.

9
FREEDOM FROM SORROW

The basic driving force behind every human action is a desire for liberation from sorrow and for the attainment of joy. Why else would a person do anything if he did not have the urge to relieve sorrow and acquire joy?

Every religion assures protection from sorrow. People are not attracted by methods that do not give such an assurance. But one might ask whether that assurance will be fulfilled or not.

Once, a pupil asked his guru, 'Sir! A great many people do religious worship, observe religious festivals, attend religious discussions and listen to spiritual discourses. But there does not appear to be any change in their lives and conduct. Why is that so?'

It is an important question indeed. It was very pertinent before and also applies to the present. It seems to be an all-time question. The same situation exists in the religious world today: people go on practising religion, but their lives remain untransformed.

The guru was a realized soul. He thought deeply into the question and said, 'It is a good question. Please do me a favour; bring me a pitcher of wine.' The pupil stood nonplussed and stared at the master's face. He could not understand what a pitcher of wine had to do with his question. The guru said, 'Get all the other pupils here.' The guru directed the pupils to have a mouthful of wine each from the pitcher and spit it out immediately. They did as they were directed. The pitcher was emptied. The guru asked, 'Does anyone feel intoxicated?' All of them spoke simultaneously, 'O master! How can it be possible? We would have been intoxicated if the wine had descended below our throats. We held the wine in our mouths only for a moment and then spat it out. It did not go down our throats. How could there be any intoxication?'

The guru asked the pupil, 'Is your question answered?'

The pupil said, 'It is not clear to me.'

The guru explained, 'Today, religion is taken up in a big way and is instantly disgorged. It does not go down our throats; it does not touch our hearts. What result do you expect then? How can our lives be transformed? Religion has its own intoxication. How is it to be dispersed? As long as the precepts of religion do not descend the throat, they cannot produce any effect. In order to make the wine of religion go down the throat, it is necessary to develop intellectual and reasoning power; a coordination of the two is necessary and this, along with direct insight, characterizes both philosophy and the philosopher.'

If the fire of true religion cannot be ignited, then it is worth investigating where the fault lies. The fault may lie in:

- The remedy.

    If the fault lies in the remedy, then another remedy should be used.

- The physician.
  If the fault lies with the physician, then another physician should be consulted.
- The method of using the remedy.
  If the fault lies in the method, then it should be changed.
- The patient himself.
  If the fault lies with the patient, then the nature of the patient needs to be refined.

Let us take these possibilities one by one:

- There does not seem to be any deficiency in the spiritual form of religion. But, being single-sided, its aspect as a cult or as a form of worship has disintegrated totally. Chanting the name of God may help achieve concentration. So will reading scriptures and practising other forms of worship. But can they help us acquire concentration if our minds are not filled with thoughts of non-violence? Can they help us attain concentration unless truth is enshrined in them? Can they promote concentration if our minds are not free of desires? Only a peaceful mind free from all desire can concentrate. The present insufficiency of religion lies in its instrumental aspect which is becoming stronger than the materialistic or the substantive aspect. This can be corrected by giving first preference to the substantive aspect and second preference to the instrumental aspect of religion.
- Most religious preceptors are dedicated not so much to religion as to a particular sect. That is why exposure to religion is more a reinforcement of tradition than a search for truth. An ordinary man can accept his incompleteness, but this is not so easy for a religious leader. A sociologist can change his former opinion in

the light of the revelation of new facts but a religious guru hesitates to do so. The difficulty for religious exponents is that they lack direct realization. A religious preceptor is one who can awaken his intuitive power through rigorous spiritual practice, who has dived deep into the ocean of knowledge. He himself is a totally transformed personality. What is expected from a religious leader is that he should pass on to his followers the knowledge gained through self-realization and intuition.

Pillars which are erected too close to each other do not permit a building to expand. At the same time, they should not be so far apart that it becomes impossible to construct a building on them. It is natural for there to be some distance between thoughts and practice. Religion is the process by which the distance between thoughts and practice can be reduced. Religion is an inner light which enlightens others. It paves the path for a smooth and happy life. The inner world is without expectations while the outer world is full of them. Bridging the gap between thought and action means moving from the world of acceptance to the world of non-acceptance, or from the synthetic approach to the analytical approach. In the world of religion, one desires to find freedom from suffering but people do not follow the practice which enables us to attain freedom. That is why religion is no longer fruitful. The only practice which can enable us to attain freedom is the practice of non-attachment and control over desire. Attachment and lack of control over desire cause suffering. No disease can be cured without removing the cause itself. Therefore, from the viewpoint of religion, it is of the utmost importance to practise the principles of non-attachment and control over one's desires. Following these principles will lead us to a happy and peaceful life.

☞ Religion has acquired a hereditary character. Consequently, a religious person adopts religion not through independent prudence or discrimination but through hereditary tradition. In former times, the son of a Vaishya and the son of a Kshatriya followed the occupations of their forefathers. Similarly, a religious person practised the religion followed by his father. Now, the tradition of hereditary occupations has changed: the son of a businessman may choose his own profession and become a doctor or an engineer. But there is still no such practice in the field of religion. I do not propound the thesis that people should not adopt the religion of their forefathers. But, before following any religion, we should analyse the religion that we are going to follow. We should check whether that religion will help us progress in spirituality and transform our consciousness.

A religious revolution demands a cleansing of the impurities in the religion. Only after such a revolution, can religion fulfil its promise of 'freedom from sorrow'.

ESSENCE

- ☞ The basic driving force behind every action is liberation from sorrow.
- ☞ Religion is the process by which the distance between thought and practice can be dissolved.
- ☞ A revolution in the way we think of religion is required to free man from sorrow.

10

SPIRITUAL JOY

This universe is a sea of vibrations. Everywhere there is a flux of vibrations. It would be a prodigious task to search out something that did not vibrate. We all know more or less about the physical waves that science teaches us about, but the vast world of psychic waves is still unknown to many. To know the hidden power working behind a human life, one should try to learn something about these waves.

THE SCIENCE OF SPIRITUAL-PSYCHIC VIBRATIONS
Human beings are subjected to four kinds of vibrations:
  i. Vibrations of the physical body
  ii. Vibrations of the vital energy
  iii. Vibrations of karma
  iv. Vibrations of the soul

Each aspect of our existence, namely the physical body, prana (vital energy), karma and consciousness, is in the form of vibrations of different gravities. The intensity of the vibrations generated by the physical body is low. The vibrations of prana are higher, those of karma still higher, while the vibrations of consciousness are the highest. A common man's experience is limited to the gross vibration of the physical body. His sensations of joy and sorrow are confined to it. As long as he lives on the level of physical consciousness, he does not have the capacity to imagine anything beyond it that is capable of giving joy.

There is no need to explain the first type—physical vibrations—because they are as easy as seeing one's reflection in a mirror. When one goes deep into subtle vibrations and understands them, the gross vibrations of the physical body do not seem important.

The second type of vibrations are those of the life-controlling force. This type is the expressive form of vibrations generated by a combination of the pure vibrations of the soul and the vibrations of karma. It determines one's lifespan, and physical as well as mental strength. The difference which we notice in the physical and mental strength of a person is due to the difference in their vital energy.

The breath also vibrates. Its vibration produces bioelectricity, the vital energy which is the controlling force of life. It is called ayussya, the life-determining prana. It vibrates and causes further vibrations in all the pranas: five sense organs, mind, speech and body. There are ten pranas. Our entire life depends on their support.

The third type of vibrations are those of the karmic body—a body which is formed as the result of a condensed form of vibrations accumulated due to previous deeds (karmas). This type of vibrations form the regulatory force of our emotions and circumstances. One way to transform these vibrations is meditation.

Each type of vibrations vibtrate in their own way. The vibrations of mohaniya karma are the thickest and the most numerous. Emotions, excitement, fear, greed, hatred—all these are vibrations of delusion. They do not cease on their own. Some of them produce joy while the others produce sorrow.

According to Jain philosophy, there are eight karmas:
- Gyanavarniya karma—the karma that obscures knowledge
- Darshanavarniya karma—the karma that obscures intuition
- Vedaniya karma—the karma that produces feelings
- Mohaniya karma—the karma that deludes
- Ayushya karma—the karma that determines the lifespan
- Naam karma—the karma that decides the build of the body
- Gotra karma—the karma that decides status
- Antaray karma—the karma that obstructs

The fourth type of vibrations are those of the consciousness, the soul, which is the ultimate pure form of existence. Pure knowledge, pure intuition and eternal bliss constitute the pure form of happiness that radiates from the soul. Sorrow is an imposed sensation which can be eliminated through meditation.

MEDITATION: A WAY TO ENHANCE JOY

What are joy and sorrow in reference to this world of vibrations? Let us understand this clearly. The feelings of joy and sorrow are dependent on various kinds of waves generated in the mind. When alpha waves emerge in the brain, one feels joy.

That is a scientific fact. A question arises here: how is this possible? This joy resides within us but we often try to find it in the outer world. This can be explained in a better way through an incident.

A young boy had recently joined a meditation camp. He always used to complain that he could not sit for more than half an hour in one place because he felt restless. One day, fortunately, his awareness turned to the centre of his intuition. He started feeling pleasant vibrations and was able to sit there like a statue for almost two hours. His family members started worrying. I went to the boy and touched his intuition centre. The boy opened his eyes and asked, 'Why have you interrupted me?' He wanted to sit there for a longer time. When he was told that he had been sitting for two hours, he explained that he had been so engrossed in inner joy that it was very difficult to come out of it. Such real happiness can be experienced through meditation.

This realization can come only when a man looks inside himself. Only then will he know that bliss exists within. It cannot be explained or conceived otherwise. True belief in religion and spirituality can exist only in that person who has realized it from the very depth of his consciousness. One has to perceive it, understand it and only then, finally, know that immense happiness lies within. A person who practises preksha dhyana achieves concentration and the restlessness of his mind starts disappearing.

When we practise meditation, our concentration power increases, due to which the alpha waves in the brain are generated rhythmically. This gives a person a great sensation of joy as compared to the one achieved by material things.

When beta and theta waves are generated in the brain, a

person feels irritated, negative thoughts are aroused within him, and he becomes sorrowful. These waves are generated when a person's consciousness resides at the physical level, that is, the material world.

These waves generated within a man make him sorrowful regardless of the fact that he may be a multimillionaire. A person experiences eternal joy regardless of any financial conditions when alpha waves are generated.

THE POWER OF MANTRAS

Thoughts, memory and imagination produce vibrations. Some of them are pleasant while others are unpleasant. Cults of devotion and the recitation of mantras are also based on the theory of vibrations. It is believed that a particular kind of sound is able to produce a certain kind of vibration. In recitation exercises, compound words are recited loudly in order to produce a certain kind of vibration. The theory behind the recitation of mantras is the theory of vibrations. The composers of the mantras knew that mantras with a particular arrangement of letters of the alphabet that was in use in ancient times would produce specific kinds of vibration. The structure of the mantra shastra is based and developed on this theory.

In ancient times, there were different methods based on the theory of vibrations to relieve one from difficult situations. That is why different devotional cults, faiths and ideologies of knowledge and action came into practice in India. Whichever path one adopted, its only aim was to produce vibrations capable of destroying unfavourable conditions.

Mantras were believed to be efficacious in increasing the energy in the body. A system of mantras was believed to bring monetary gains. There were preventive mantras to ward off future calamities, others to treat disease, to produce joy and to destroy grief. Sound could produce vibrations which, in turn, could change the course of natural events. Different kinds of idols also induce vibrations. Such vibrations are produced through meditation.

When these vibrations were properly investigated, it resulted in the development of various kinds of theories. Vibrations could be stopped by an opposite kind of vibrations. Bhavana—a repetitive suggestion of a particular thought—is one of the means of producing vibrations to enter subtle experiences. A lot can be achieved by producing counter-vibrations.

It is quite pertinent to ask: if the vibrations of hunger could be subdued by counter-vibrations then why should we eat in order to satisfy our hunger? This seems quite a natural and logical question. It should be remembered, however, that the theory of counter-vibrations is applicable only on the level of consciousness. Some vibrations affect the body or the pudgala (matter) while others have a psychological application. For example, vibrations caused by delusion are concerned only with consciousness. Vibrations of karma which produce auspicious as well as inauspicious feelings affect only the pudgala. Hunger cannot be quenched by producing counter-vibrations but delusions can be removed.

The theory of counter-vibrations has been developed in the field of spiritual practice. Practitioners are called upon to perceive and know the vibrations which will result in producing counter-vibrations of hatred, grief, anger, etc.

JOY: A FUSION OF ENERGY

Vibrations connected with craving are carnal vibrations, and can be subdued by counter-vibrations. Some vibrations are connected with the enjoyment of external objects while others are connected with internal or spiritual joy. The electrical energy which resides in the brain produces carnal vibrations. When this energy flows downwards, it produces materialistic pleasure. It is necessary to understand that this materialistic pleasure is temporary in nature. But, it is only these vibrations which are responsible for the sense of pleasure. Also, these vibrations can be produced artificially.

In order to generate the counter-vibrations that oppose them, we have to carry the descending energy upwards. This needs a lot of control. The electricity which resides in the brain is positive energy while the electricity which resides in the centre connected to carnal drives is negative. When vital energy begins to flow into the sahasrar chakra—the centre of knowledge—it produces vibrations which are congenial to one's self. We experience a joy never felt before. As compared to this joy, the pleasures born of carnal vibrations are insignificant. One who has risen to the level of spiritual experience will never wish to relinquish it. He will remain self-absorbed for hours and hours together and will not feel dejected even when the state of spiritual experience comes to an end. On the other hand, he feels much more exhilarated and stronger.

People often ask: what is joy? Joy implies the transformation of negative energy into positive. The next question that arises is how exactly does this happen? It happens when the negative energy of the centres which are connected to the carnal drives reaches the positive centre of knowledge, that is, the centre of the brain. This fusion produces extraordinary vibrations.

Knowledge and consciousness originate in the human nervous system. Consciousness pervades the entire body. The portion of the body which extends from the lower end of the spinal column to the brain is the chief centre of consciousness. It is in this area that consciousness manifests itself. This is also the origin of chita, mind, sense organs, feelings, counter-feelings, and knowledge. They find expression in this area only. It is the storehouse of energy, and also the centre of the sensory and motor nerves.

Man knows how to push his energy downwards but he does not know how to push it upwards. The same energy which is flowing downwards can be directed upwards. The downward flow of energy from the brain implies man's entry into the material world. The upward flow of energy from the centre connected to the carnal drives implies man's entry into the spiritual world. The latter gives us a taste of spiritual joy. These feelings are conditioned by the direction towards which energy is flowing. The upward flow has been termed internal enjoyment or love of 'the self'.

The vital force which flows downwards causes the death of spiritual life, but when it begins to flow upwards it brings life. Once a person masters the art of channelizing the flow of energy, he begins his journey on the ascending path of life. This ascending path leads to the progress of the real self, the soul. This ascent is arrested as long as the vital energy remains confined to the lower parts of the body. In the state of the rising of energy, the consciousness from the sushumna channel—a path in the spinal column in which vital energy flows—rises to the centre of the brain and arrives at the stage of pure knowledge and self-realization. The sushumna channel and the sahasrar chakra are two powerful centres in the body. Experienced practitioners attach great importance to them. When our faith in spiritual joy develops, we begin to feel the vibrations in the psyche which are vibrations of positive energy.

SPIRITUAL JOY

Somebody asked Lord Mahavira, 'What do we achieve from religious faith?' Lord Mahavira replied, 'Religious faith puts an end to all kinds of curiosity.'

When spiritual vibrations begin, the curiosity about the material vibrations comes to an end. One of the methods to stop curiosity about the centre connected to the carnal drives is to push up the energy collected there. Practitioners have to resolve and pull upwards the muscles of the area known as apana (anus), which is located at the lower end of the spinal column. If this is done for fifteen to twenty minutes or for half an hour, the vibration that produces spiritual joy will begin.

The electricity in the tongue is negative while the one in the head is positive. If you touch your palate with your tongue, then you feel a strange pleasure, which will produce in you a state of self-absorption. The fusion of positive and negative charges of energy produces a spiritual vibration. Material vibrations keep on disappearing gradually as the spiritual vibrations become intense. It appears to the practitioner as if he were entering the most valuable experience.

The subject we have discussed is not a matter of argument. It refers to experience. Mere explanation cannot take the practitioner to the depths of experience. He has to practise and exert himself to attain the experience. He may face difficulties while doing this exercise. At times, his progress may come to a standstill. However, there is only one path which leads to all desired ends.

Material pleasures cannot compete with the joys of the spiritual world. The discussion about the joy of the spiritual world may appear attractive but may also create doubts in the minds of listeners who may begin to weigh one alternative against the other. Language is not a very efficient tool even if it is used by the one who has perfect knowledge—even tirthankars—and may produce doubts. The testing ground for both faith and scepticism is experience. There is no other way. The only aim of sadhana is to enable the practitioner to feel the vibrations discussed and to make him realize that spiritual joy is not dependent upon agencies which are external to the soul.

One who acquires knowledge of the internal vibrations can also know the external vibrations. It is true the other way, too. He may not become interested in internal vibrations until he has known the external vibrations. He comes to realize that the former are more joy-giving and profitable.

ESSENCE

- All the hidden power working in our lives is in the form of waves.
- Joy and sorrow both depend upon the waves generated in the brain.
- Positive vibrations generated through meditation can transform the negative vibrations.
- The fusion of positive and negative charges of energy produces spiritual vibrations.

11

SELF-REALIZATION: A STEP TOWARDS A HAPPY LIFE

When people come to me, they generally introduce themselves as doctor, engineer, lawyer, collector, and so on. But no one tells me that he knows his soul. Their introduction is related either to their qualification or their business but not related to the self. It includes only worldly affairs. This is the root cause of sorrow. A person always wants to know about others but never tries to know about his own self. This ignorance creates a problem not only for him but also for others. In this problem-driven age, if he wants to make an attempt to find a solution, he has to change his path from a materialistic life to focusing upon his own self.

If we consider matters from a non-absolute point of view, we see that knowledge of the materialistic life is both important and necessary. But if one knows only about the external world and does not pay any attention to the self, his sorrow will go on increasing.

SELF-REALIZATION AND FREEDOM FROM SORROW

The question is: 'How can we recognize our own selves?' This is the biggest question of the modern age. Even the introduction includes details only about one's external qualities. People often introduce themselves as 'I am a professor', 'I am a Member of Parliament', 'I am a poet', and so on, but one never says, 'I am a common man, and am learning about religion and spirituality.' In my opinion, the happiest man on the earth is one who

- knows himself;
- is not taken in by any circumstances;
- is not influenced by favourable or unfavourable conditions;
- has conquered his ego;
- does not get frustrated by any situation.

The one who goes beyond the causes of sorrow never falls into problems. But it is difficult for anyone to be free of sorrow.

Once a man visited a holy man and said, 'Oh holy man! I am in search of truth and want to achieve eternal happiness. Please show me the right path.' The holy man replied, 'First you have to do me a favour. I am in need of a shirt. Get it for me from a person who has never experienced sorrow.'

The man left at once, thinking it would be an easy task. He set out in search of it and arrived at a village. There he met a wealthy landlord and thought that he would be the right person. He said, 'I am in search of a shirt for a holy man. Can you please provide me with one? But there is only one condition—the holy man wants a shirt from a family in which no one has been unhappy.' The landlord replied, 'But I am the unhappiest person in this world. Though I have a lot of wealth, my sorrows seem to have no end. It has been six years since my first wife died. My second wife also expired due to an incurable disease.

Now, I live all alone. Continuous disputes have been going on between me and my brother. Even my two sons live away from me. Now, tell me how can I be a happy person?'

Being unsuccessful, the man moved farther in search of a happy family. For one long week, he searched thoroughly in the village but could not find a family where all the members were happy. He found that all of them were filled with sadness and unhappiness and were suffering from problems and illness. Finally, being unsuccessful in his attempts, he returned to the holy man and said, 'I was unable to complete the task given by you as your condition couldn't be fulfilled. I also came to know that nobody in this world is happy, no matter whether he is rich or poor.' The holy man said, 'You asked me about the path to eternal happiness, but now you must have realized that no one can find happiness in a materialistic life. One is continuously involved in one problem or another. A materialistic life never allows a person to live in peace. His wants and desires go on increasing. If you want to achieve eternal happiness, you will have to renounce the material world.'

Nowadays, I frequently see the newspapers flooded with news of suicide cases. Many officers end their lives because they are denied promotion, many businessmen die due to the failure of the market, students due to fear of their examination results. The increasing number of army officers committing suicide has become an issue for the government. What is the reason behind it? The reason is the absence of self-realization. In this modern age, everyone is engaged in the search for possessions. But one cannot achieve happiness through possessions. One who wants to attain real happiness has to search for truth. The truth will allow him to come out of the whirlpool of sorrow.

It seems unrealistic to say that there is no joy in the material world. There is joy, indeed, but it is momentary. A person may feel happy on buying a new house, a car and so on. But the joy achieved by these is not permanent. Money, by nature, is fickle. Its absence causes sorrow, its presence results in joy. It comes and it goes.

In spite of knowing these facts, man chases money. This will continue because money gives him a lot. It gives him material possessions which can have a deleterious effect on man's thinking. It is not possible to lead a social life without these possessions. It is not possible to completely restrict their consumption but it is essential to know their real nature. Consume an object with a detached mind so that its absence does not cause sorrow. If you are able to develop this kind of mentality, then material things will not make you happy or unhappy.

KNOWING THE SELF

When a man goes in search of truth and eternal happiness, it is necessary for him to know 'THE SELF'. It is also important for him to ask, 'WHO AM I?' As long as he doesn't know the self, various favourable and unfavourable circumstances will continue to influence him at every step of his life. Without knowing the self he cannot practise equanimity in his life. Material possessions make a man's mind fickle and unstable. In our society, we come across people who used to be polite and good-natured, but in whose behaviour a rapid change is noticed with an increase in their wealth. There are also people who are not wealthy but whose politeness and pleasant behaviour capture the hearts of many. These people understand well the ups and downs of life, but are not affected by them.

It is necessary to understand that material possessions will **not remain permanently with us.** Moreover, there is only a transitory union between material objects. That is why an object cannot give permanent happiness. Self-realization is necessary for eternal happiness. No power in the world can deprive you of happiness which is caused by self-realization. Thus, the key to eternal happiness is in our hands. No support is required from any object to feel happy. It is our outlook which creates sorrow or joy. A positive outlook is enough to lead a happy life. 'Who am I?' This question should strike your mind, again and again. The day your self-realization starts, you will get on the path to eternal happiness. Breath is the first window through which you can perceive the soul. It is by passing through this window that the journey towards the self begins. It is a journey within you. It is a journey towards self-perception. We are accustomed to looking outwards. It is the nature of the mind to run only towards the external world. Breath is the first door through which you have to enter before the journey begins. When the mind begins to follow the in-going breath, we begin to enter into our being. Breath is the soul. The body is the soul. The mind is the soul. We can reach the fag end of our journey only through them.

It is a delusion to want to see the soul directly. The soul, which is the supreme reality, the supreme existence and the subtlest entity, cannot be an object of perception by the gross sense organs. To say so is a big mistake.

To say that we should try to see the soul through the soul means that first, we should engage the mind in perceiving the vibrations of breath. Second, it means engaging the mind in perceiving the vibrations of the body and the sensations. Third, it means watching one's own thought process. Once you have travelled through these three stages, you will encounter the aura around the body and get a chance to perceive it.

The atmosphere in which we live is full of vibrations. Those who have happened to see the aura have felt that, while doing so, they were floating in an ocean of vibrations whose expanse they were unable to imagine. After seeing the aura we will be able to come in contact with the vital force. It is the vital energy which is the source of internal and external vibrations. It is the vital energy which immerses breath, mind and body into the soul so that they become the soul. The mind which comes in contact with the life force and becomes permeated with it becomes alive and part and parcel of the soul. When the vital force achieves a relationship with the mind, the mind becomes activated. The vital force, when it gets associated with the breath, activates the latter. Breath begins to vibrate because of this association. It is the vital energy which makes the heart throb, the breath vibrate, the mental process begin, and the spectrum of aura radiate. The ever-flowing stream of consciousness is the source of vital energy. Vital energy inducts life through the entire body and transforms everything which is non-soul into consciousness. Breath is the first stage in the process of sadhana which culminates in the perception of the soul.

ESSENCE

- Self-realization is the first step towards happiness. The habit of knowing others but not oneself is the root cause of sorrow.
- Real happiness can be achieved through realization of the eternal truth.
- The joy given by material possessions is unrealistic and momentary.
- For eternal happiness it is essential to know 'THE SELF', and to ask the question, again and again, 'WHO AM I?'

12

WHO AM I?

From time immemorial, man has faced the question, 'Who am I?' This important question has been endlessly contemplated upon. Thousands of men in spiritual pursuit have repeatedly asked the question. Many of them after years of pursuit have reached the core of their being and finally resolved it. Maharshi Raman often reiterated endlessly, 'Who am I? Who am I?'

Here I will go deep into the topic from an entirely different angle. Do I really have to know who I am? Can't I, for a moment, completely set aside the question of whether I am soul or God? Is it possible to ask this question purely in relation to the body? Am I an iccha-purush, a person who is dominated by desire? Am I a prana-purush, a person possessed of abundant vitality? Am I a pragya-purush, a person in possession of great wisdom? I do not need to go far to seek an answer. I don't have to read any book either. I don't need to do anything. Let me just observe in what part of the body I usually reside and I shall know who I am. It will be crystal clear by itself.

The body can be divided into three parts:
- The part between the top of the brain and the throat
- The part between the throat and the navel
- The part below the navel

The diligent seeker must locate the centre of his consciousness in one of these three parts. He must ask himself, 'Does my consciousness abide in the part of the body above or below the navel?' Those centres where one's consciousness resides the most will be the most active. If consciousness moves below the navel, then the lower centres will get activated. If consciousness stays longer in the part above the navel, then the centres in that sphere will be charged with energy. The centres located in the part where consciousness abides the least will become inactive; the centres where it dwells the most will be rejuvenated.

When the centres are deprived of the nourishment offered by consciousness, they get depleted of energy, become lethargic and dormant. All we need to know clearly is the answer to the question, 'Where am I?' We need to be clear about where we are. In which of the three parts of the body do we wander the most? The moment that is clear, we shall know who we are.

ICCHA-PURUSH

The navel is the source of the awakening of desires; all cravings are centred there. It is the source of attachment and restlessness, of lewdness and immorality. Desires are born there. Consciousness gets repeatedly stuck there. Consequently, the centre gets activated. There is a deluge of cravings, waves of lewdness, incessantly rising desires which clearly indicate that I am an iccha-purush. Cravings are dominant there. Yearnings are innumerable and beyond control.

A person whose consciousness resides below the navel is

known as an iccha-purush. This type of person is always inclined towards the material world. His desires are unlimited. In order to fulfil his desires, he indulges in immoral activities. And yet, his desires are never fulfilled. Consequently, he is filled with anger and jealousy. He gets frustrated and often thinks of putting an end to his life.

PRANA-PURUSH

A person whose consciousness lies between the throat and the navel is termed as a prana-purush. Such a person masters the art of self-control or restraint. His actions are centred on his needs and not on desires. In other words, his desires are limited to his needs. This can be explained through a story.

Once, a king wanted to appoint a new minister. So he summoned all the talented men of his kingdom to arrive at 4 a.m. sharp at his court. The passage to his court was decorated magnificently. There were a number of shops filled with eye catching goods, such as gold, silver, diamonds, rubies, and so on. Not only this, there were also stalls displaying the best delicacies from all over the country. There was a constant announcement being made, 'Today, you can take any of these items without paying for them.'

This was too tempting an offer to resist. Most of the candidates got lured and stopped at more than one stall. They got entangled in those attractions and started collecting the precious items. They all seemed to have forgotten the real reason for their being there. Only one man did not stop at any of the stalls but headed straight toward the king's chamber. He was able to reach there at 4 a.m. sharp.

The king was surprised and asked the young man, 'You

reached here on time. Weren't you tempted by the things in any of the stalls?' The man replied politely, 'Sir, I had come here to meet you. Though I was attracted by the offers, I practised self-control and remained focused on my objective of meeting you.'

The king said, 'A person who has developed the virtue of self-restraint can attain anything in his life.' The man was appointed as minister.

This can happen only when a person's consciousness resides between the throat and the navel—his desires will remain under control.

PRAGYA-PURUSH

A person whose consciousness flows between the top of the head and the throat is known as a pragya-purush. He always remains in a blissful state. Although he lives in the material world like any other man, his outlook is spiritual. His consciousness is enlightened by the light of intuition. He has controlled his emotions and passions. He remains uninfluenced by the outer circumstances.

Once, a yogi was meditating under a huge banyan tree on the outskirts of a village. A group of shepherds had come there to graze their cattle. One of them noticed a big black cobra climbing on to the yogi's body. He called the other shepherds and they were all frightened. When the yogi completed his meditation, they gathered around him. One of them bowed and asked, 'A few minutes ago, a venomous cobra had climbed up your body. Didn't you realize it? Weren't you frightened?' The yogi smiled and said, 'Oh child! I was with my soul at that time. I didn't experience the sensations of my physical body.' Such is the condition of a man whose consciousness lies in the top of the head. The pragya-purush becomes so tuned to his inner self that insecurities and fear cease to disturb him. He always remains calm and positive.

ANALYSE YOURSELF

If your desires are unlimited and passions are uncontrolled, then your consciousness is roaming below the navel. You can recognize yourself as an iccha-purush, a person with preponderant desires.

If your desires are limited, your consciousness of restraining from material things is awakened, you will realize that your consciousness is centred between the navel and the throat. You will recognize yourself as a person of preponderant vitality and can categorize yourself as a prana-purush.

If you are detached from worldly desires and you have the power to subdue your emotions, then you realize that your consciousness stays up between the top of the head and the throat. You will be a person possessed with preponderant wisdom; you will become a pragya-purush.

If you are an iccha-purush, you will lead a sorrowful life. If you are a prana-purush, then you will lead a happy life. But if you are a pragya-purush, then you will remain in a blissful state forever.

When consciousness is active in the upper regions, it awakens the higher centres, and the lower centres get deactivated. When consciousness is active in the upper sphere, desire itself will work in a disciplined manner. The really important thing is to locate the control centres in one's body.

A woman was driving at a furious speed. A police van chased her and the policeman said, 'It's a crime to drive so fast.' The woman cried, 'I know but I am helpless. The controlling device has gone out of hand. I don't even remember where it is located.' She rushed along, collided with a tree and died on the spot.

When the controlling device gets out of order it foreshadows instant annihilation. The vehicle of life glides smoothly as long as the controlling device and the brakes function normally. When the controlling device breaks down, one finds oneself confronted by danger.

There are innumerable control centres in the body. The brain is the controller, the regulator of them all. The nervous system and the spinal cord (sushumna) are the control centres. The man who has experienced the movement of consciousness in his sushumna or in his brain or in the various parts of the body, including front and back, right and left, and in the upper regions, is already in possession of many great secrets. There is one controlling centre in the upper part of the body, one at the back, one each on the right and the left, and one in the middle. It is possible to make our body transparent at these five junctions. Our whole body constitutes a magnetic field but it is possible to make it more magnetic at these five points. When it is fully magnetic, clairvoyance is born.

As long as consciousness is turned outwards we cannot achieve happiness. When consciousness is turned inwards, only then can one achieve the state of joy.

ESSENCE

- All types of cravings have their origin in the navel.
- A person whose consciousness resides between the throat and the navel can control his desires.
- Trying to direct consciousness towards the upper centre is to achieve the true state of joy.

MEDITATION: PERCEPTION OF BREATHING

1. POSTURE:
Select a posture in which you can sit comfortably and continuously for forty-five minutes—full lotus, half lotus, cross-legged or diamond.

2. MUDRAS—THE POSITION OF THE HANDS (ANY ONE):
   i. Gyana Mudra:
      Place your right hand on the right knee and the left on the left knee, palms turned up. Touch the tip of the thumb with the tip of the index finger with a slight pressure. Keep the other fingers straight and relaxed.
   ii. Brahma Mudra:
      Place both hands on your lap, one above the other, palms turned up, the left palm under the right one. Keep your eyes softly closed.

3. RECITATION OF MAHAPRANA DHVANI:
   - Keep your lips softly closed, your spinal column and neck straight, without stiffness.

- Inhale deeply and silently for about four to five seconds with a calm mind, empty of thoughts, all muscles relaxed.
- Concentrate on the top of your head.
- Keeping your lips closed, exhale slowly, making the sound of mmm ……… through the nostrils, like the buzzing of a bee.
- This may last eight to ten seconds. Inhale again and keep repeating this exercise for five minutes.

4. **KAYOTSARGA (RELAXATION):**
   - Relax all the muscles in your body.
   - Release all the stress from your body.
   - Concentrate and allow your mind to travel, taking a trip to all the parts of your body, from the big toe of your right foot to the top of the head.
   - Give an auto-suggestion to each and every muscle to relax and feel it relaxing.
   - Concentrate deeply and remain completely alert.

5. **LONG BREATHING:**
   - Direct full attention to your breathing. Regulate it: make it slow, deep and rhythmic. Focus your full attention on the navel and become fully aware of the contraction and expansion of the abdomen, accompanying each exhalation and inhalation respectively.
   - Continue the perception of the navel region for about five minutes until the breath has been

MEDITATION: PERCEPTION OF BREATHING

regulated to a slow rhythm.
- Continuing the slow, deep and rhythmic breathing, shift your attention from the navel and focus it inside the nostrils, at the junction where the two nostrils meet. Be fully aware of each and every breath.
- Maintain the continuity of awareness throughout the session.

6. **ALTERNATE BREATHING:**
   - Close your right nostril with your thumb, inhale slowly through your left nostril for five seconds. At the end of the inhalation, close the left nostril with your index finger, release your right nostril and exhale slowly for five seconds.
   - At the end of the exhalation, without pausing, begin to inhale through the right nostril. Inhale for five seconds.
   - Now close the right nostril and release the left one and exhale slowly through the left nostril for five seconds. Complete the exhalation. This completes the first round since the original starting point has been reached.
   - Without interruption, repeat and perform the exercise for several rounds. Try to maintain the rhythm.

Conclude the meditation session by chanting the mahaprana dhvani three times.

13

WHO IS THE HAPPIEST MAN?

Who is the richest person in the world? Which celebrity owns the most expensive house? Who has presented his wife with the most precious gift? We are usually interested in finding the answers to such questions and comparing the statistics. Even the newspapers are filled with such surveys. But have we ever tried to make a survey of more important matters? Have we ever asked the question, 'Which country houses the most honest people?' Or, 'Which country has made efforts to develop moral values in its citizens?'

Let me ask a similar question here: 'Who is the happiest person in the world?' There may be many answers to this question. A person living in the material world would say, 'One who owns a lot of wealth is the happiest man.' Or he may say, 'The person who enjoys a lot of power and luxuries can be considered the happiest.'

This is a myth. An individual may have a big bungalow, many cars, numerous properties and a well-established business but he is still unable to sleep. He tries hard to get sound sleep but is unable to do so. He needs medication to sleep. Can we call him the 'happiest person'?

CHARACTERISTICS OF A HAPPY PERSON

The first characteristic of a happy person is the ability to sleep peacefully and wake up peacefully. Today, a large segment of the population is dependent upon medication to sleep. There was a time when people used to sleep early and wake up early in the morning in the Brahma muhurta. One who wakes up in the Brahma muhurta is free of many kinds of illness and enjoys mental peace.

Today lifestyles have changed completely. People start working at ten in the night and stop at four in the morning. This has disturbed the system which has been prevalent from ancient times.

One who relies on medication for sleep cannot be called happy. All yogis wake up in the Brahma muhurta. My guru, Acharyashree Tulsi, always used to get up at 4 a.m. and I have followed that practice in the past six decades. Even at the age of ninety, I still have the habit of getting up in the Brahma muhurta.

Nowadays, people are in the habit of sleeping late and getting up late. A mother was trying to get her son out of bed. She said, 'Open your eyes. Look, the sun has risen so high.' The son, unwilling to get up, said, 'How can you compare me to the sun? It can get up early because it goes to bed early. I always go to bed late.'

The new generation has found many excuses for its unhealthy sleeping habits. Many of them feel that their working efficiency increases much more in the night. According to

UNDERSTANDING JOY AND SORROW

science, the secretion of the hormone melatonin starts at 4 a.m. and continues till sunrise. It keeps man fresh and energetic throughout the day. This coincides with the period of the Brahma muhurta.

The second characteristic of a happy person is the power to restrain personal consumption. The greed for consuming more makes a man restless. The limitless use of material things and the attachment to them gives rise to stress. In the present scenario of the stock market, the rise and fall in the prices of stocks results in the rise and fall of stress in brokers and traders. In ancient times, people betting in speculation could not live a peaceful life; the same thing applies today.

The utility of wealth cannot be denied, but blind attachment to it and its limitless accumulation by the wealthy affect the life of the common man. A simple person in a village is generally much more satisfied and happier than a city-dweller who actually has many more options for living a comfortable life. Unnecessary use of money for one's pleasure becomes the cause of sorrow for oneself and others. But still, the attraction towards material pleasures is increasing day by day. Unnecessary travelling just for the sake of entertainment has increased hugely. The increase in the price of petrol and diesel has not affected the number of vehicles on the road. Even when a person already owns a number of cars, he is tempted to buy a new one. He becomes restless until he achieves his objective. In this situation, how can we even imagine that the possession of objects brings happiness? Happiness does not lie in material comforts; it lies in living a restrained life. This restrained life may appear difficult but bliss exists within. Such happiness is beyond the power of expression.

There is no way other than restraint for attaining happiness. **No scientist in the world can invent an apparatus** for producing happiness. Happiness is a by-product of restraint and satisfaction. Nowhere in the world can an abundance of material posessions without contentment give happiness.

Our ancestors lived a simple life with limited comforts. They lived in thatched huts, ate simple food, wore simple clothes, and were happy and satisfied. At present, in spite of having abundant facilities, we are not as happy. This makes it clear that a restrained life is a happy life, in the true sense.

The third characteristic of a happy person is his capability to limit the use of his wealth, not because he is a miser but because he is content. Many people who practise penance or fast often feel an inner bliss. A person who has surplus luxuries but does not use them realizes that happiness lies not in using them but restraining from them.

The fourth characteristic of a happy person is that he thinks not only about the present or the future but also about the final result. Those who do not think about the final results of their acts will come to regret them at some point of time, like the woman whose story I am going to relate.

Once, in a village, a woman lived with her only son. He came home one day with some pencils and erasers. When his mother inquired about them, he said that he liked them and was able to slip them away quietly from his classmate. The mother did not say anything but just smiled. The next day, the boy managed to steal a few more items from another classmate. The mother merely appreciated her son's ability to do it and the skill that made him successful in his plans. The habit of stealing grew day by day. As he became older, he began to bring home expensive things. His stealing progressed from school to the neighbourhood, and so on. The mother ignored her son's habit and he eventually grew to be a notorious gangster.

His terror spread far and wide. The police began to hunt for him all over the country. Finally, they managed to arrest him and presented him before the court. The court decided to hang him for the endless list of his crimes. He was asked for his last wish. The thief said that he had only one wish and that was to see his mother. The court granted it. When his mother came to see him, the thief immediately took a knife and chopped off her nose. The mother was shocked by her son's behaviour. The thief then said, 'If you had slapped me on my first act of stealing or had tried to correct my mistake in my childhood, then I would not have had to see this day. It is because of you that I am going to be hanged today. You did not care to see the outcome of your actions. So, you deserve this.'

That is what happens when one does not think of the outcome of one's actions. It is necessary for a person to do so if he wants to lead a happy life.

A question arises here: 'From where does misery come?' Misery does not come from anywhere, it is man who generates it. There is no factory manufacturing sorrow. I have visited many cities like Ahmedabad, Mumbai, etc. Wherever I went, I asked people, 'Is there any factory manufacturing sorrow or joy? If one exists, I would like to see it.' Nobody could answer me. Man himself generates sorrow or misery within him because he does not ponder on the results of his actions.

The fifth characteristic of a happy man is the capacity to think. One reason for lack of joy is that man does not know how to think rationally. Thoughts do not stay for a long time in a sorrowful mind. He starts to think about one thing and soon switches over to another. A man's nature is known from his thoughts. The level of his happiness can also be ascertained through his thoughts. **Only a happy man can think in a sound manner.**

WHO IS THE HAPPIEST MAN?

Let us consider what is meant by sound thinking. Once, Acharya Bhikshu was sitting alone under a tree. A few people passing by asked him who he was. Acharya Bhikshu told them that he was a monk and his name was Bhikhan. The men began to wonder if he was the same man being praised everywhere. They had drawn a different image of him in their minds. They had imagined him to be a highly impressive personality surrounded by a crowd of followers. Seeing him by himself and very modest, they fell into a dilemma. Acharya Bhikshu showed no concern over what the men were thinking about him because his mind was fully composed. He cared neither for praise nor for blame. He did not believe in pomp or show. People had a high regard for him because of his simplicity and modesty.

A man with good thoughts is respected everywhere and remains happy.

It is very difficult to achieve happiness in life. Though a man might collect materials for his comfort, it is not within his control to be happy. Generally, the affluent class has no dearth of material comforts but there are very few who actually feel happy. Most of them suffer from tension and sorrow. They are not content with what they have. They continue to be unhappy thinking of what they don't have. So they go on amassing material wealth and comforts and, in the process, they fail to enjoy the comforts they have. The sorrow of negativism always troubles them.

Shekhsadi was a reputed holy man. One day, he saw a lame beggar who seemed quite happy and satisfied. The beggar's face had no signs of worry. Observing him, he contemplated his own self and thought, 'In spite of being a holy man and thinker, I remain gloomy throughout the day, while this beggar is totally content despite leading a materially bankrupt life, deprived of even the barest necessities. Although he is disabled, he is happy and at ease. I have almost everything with me, but I am unhappy while the beggar who has nothing is happy. What is his secret?'

Shekhsadi went to the beggar and asked, 'You are so deprived, how is it that you are still happy?'

The beggar replied, 'I have learnt the philosophy of never brooding over the negative things of life. I always thank God who has blessed me with a healthy mind. I remain happy because of it and never feel sad about my disability.'

Shekhsadi grasped the secret of his happiness.

There are two kinds of people—the ones who focus on what they do not have and the ones who focus on what they have. Those who keep brooding over what they don't have remain unhappy despite having uncountable luxuries. They are called pessimists. Those who appreciate the things they have, in spite of having nothing much, are called optimists.

Human psychology categorizes people into pessimists and optimists.

In today's world, pessimists are in abundance. A millionaire compares himself to a person wealthier than him, and he thinks that he needs more wealth. Thereafter, he keeps accumulating wealth at the cost of happiness. Similarly, a person with great wealth keeps worrying and comparing himself to others who are better off materially. In the process, he remains worried, restless and unhappy. Even God cannot help such greedy people.

Bliss is experienced by one who rejoices in what he has and who never worries about what he does not possess. A person who is content will never worry about what he does not possess. This kind of person remains satisfied forever, content with what he has, and is full of bliss.

ESSENCE

- The first characteristic of a happy person is an ability to sleep peacefully and wake up peacefully.
- The second is the ability to restrain personal consumption.
- The third is a limited use of his wealth.
- The fourth is living and thinking in the present.
- The fifth is sound thinking.

14

HAPPINESS THROUGH CONTEMPLATION

There are two paths in life—that of materialism and that of spiritualism. We have to understand spirituality from different perspectives. Unless a man develops the right view towards material objects he cannot be truly spiritual.

MATERIALISM

Man has an unfortunate tendency to treat material objects as permanent. He may profess to consider them as being impermanent, but in deed, in practice and in his innermost feelings, he deals with them as if they were everlasting. This is the foremost reason why the loss of any material object results in sorrow. Sorrow occurs because of attachment to material things.

As long as this attitude towards material objects remains, man cannot invoke his spiritual consciousness; he will continue to seek refuge in materialism. This shows that he is a captive of the material world. Until and unless this illusion is completely destroyed, spirituality cannot evolve.

Unfortunately, a man identifies himself totally with his body. Spirituality cannot exist until and unless matter and consciousness, that is, body and soul, are seen as different entities. The belief that 'I am different from my body' and that 'I am solitary' guides us towards spirituality.

There are four steps to realizing spirituality:
- Contemplation of impermanence.
- Contemplation of the state of 'asharana'—a state in which a person does not seek shelter.
- Contemplation of the separation of self from the material body.
- Contemplation of solitariness.

He, whose consciousness of impermanence, of asharana, of separation from the material body and of solitariness is awakened, becomes spiritual. By practising the above fourfold process, he can realize his true self.

CONTEMPLATION OF IMPERMANENCE

The practice of contemplating the impermanence of matter is the first step towards the realization of spirituality. As this practice develops, the happiness and sorrow associated with objects starts dissipating. According to our mental and emotional states, an undesired object gives us sorrow while a desired object gives us happiness. But, in the foremost state of impermanence, there is no sorrow. When the truth about acquisition and separation is completely understood, and the consciousness awakens with full realization, then there is no fear of old age and no fear of death. Only a truly spiritual person can overcome this suffering.

Merely being a leader or a preacher cannot help transcend this suffering. Only a person who lives spiritually can overcome it and enjoy continuous and infinite bliss. The one who does not realize this bliss at present can never achieve it later. Moksha is obviously achieved by one who experiences emancipation at the present moment. The practice and contemplation of impermanence is imperative for getting elevated to that realization. The practice should be so rigorous that realization actually occurs. Only that philosophy which is actually lived out during realization is considered perfect. The mere chanting of mantras will not help until it is actually realized through practice. Similarly, realizing the impermanence of matter is necessary: it is the first step towards spirituality. A spiritual person may be defined as one who has witnessed impermanence.

CONTEMPLATION OF THE STATE OF ASHARANA

The second element is asharana. King Shrenik, on seeing the young Anathi Muni, asked him, 'How did you become an ascetic at such a young age?' The ascetic replied, 'I was insecure and did not find any refuge.' Shrenik said, 'Well, I will provide you with shelter. Come. Live with me in my palace.' The ascetic said, 'O king! You yourself are insecure and still you wish to provide me with shelter? How can you become my refuge and give me true shelter?' The king was surprised and asked, 'How am I insecure? If I am the ruler of such a big empire how can I be insecure?' The ascetic said, 'O king! I was the son of a wealthy father and faced no lack of any kind. Once, I had an unbearable pain in my eye and nobody was there to share the pain. That helpless state of sickness and intense pain awakened the consciousness of asharana in me. I realized that there is no one in the world who can provide me with shelter. I am born without it. The external material world cannot provide relief and shelter. Therefore, I sought shelter within myself. With determination, the pain disappeared. The consciousness of asharana guided me towards the path of seeking true shelter and I became an ascetic. I no longer crave for anybody's shelter.'

A spiritual person is one whose consciousness of asharana is awakened.

There are two kind of persons—external seekers and internal seekers. A spiritual person is an internal seeker. An external seeker is materialistic because he is always inclined to seek externally. He searches for the solution to everything in the material world. He always yearns for objects. It is natural for anyone to move in the direction of the things towards which he is inclined. If his tendency is to seek within, then, he will surely seek the solution to everything in his spirit. Seeking internally is to seek inside the soul. This is a very simple definition of spirituality. In the state of consciousness of impermanence, any external attachment or delusion will be resolved automatically.

CONTEMPLATION OF THE SEPARATION OF SELF FROM THE MATERIAL BODY

Man has a deep attachment to his physical body. He spends a lot of time caring for it. His delusion is so profound and deep that he has accepted the body and the soul to be one and the same. His body is his only personality, and because of that, he cannot materialize his spirituality. One should practise the philosophy of contemplating over the separation of soul from the body and arrive at the knowledge that one's existence is separate from the body. When the knowledge of separation of soul from the body awakens, then spirituality starts taking root. Man accepts three traits of his personality—memory, imagination and thinking power. All these are mechanical, none of them is related to the soul. Sensation is related to the soul, it is not mechanical. Spirituality commences only when the consciousness of separation from the body awakens.

CONTEMPLATION OF SOLITARINESS

It is ironical that the more man is attached to material possessions, the more he considers himself capable, thinking that possession is strength. He does not want to be alone; that is why he keeps on complaining, 'I have done so much for my family but they have all deceived me. I have helped and cooperated with them in all circumstances but, today, they have become my worst enemies.' I really pity such people. Man experiences misery and restlessness only when he is attached and does not know the art of living by himself. No matter how kind we may be to others, how much we may help others, we should never forget that, eventually, we are alone. A person associated with this ultimate truth never experiences sorrow or misery.

The last step towards spirituality is to be solitary. Lord Mahavira attached great importance to the state of solitariness. Meditation in solitude is considered highly important. A person who learns to be solitary even while living among the crowd has learnt to lead a life free of tension. This is the truth and the essence of spirituality. Spirituality does not mean living in physical loneliness, which is achieved by renouncing society and living in a secluded place. The biggest philosophy of successful living is to realize solitude while living among people.

The causes of mental tension arising in the family and the community can be sought within this fourfold truth. Tension generally arises when a man faces an unpleasant situation. A father expects his son to take care of him in his old age. But, when he becomes old, the son cuts off the relationship and separates from him. The father becomes tense and restless, and his life becomes a burden to him.

Only those who have achieved these four truths can have a spiritual personality. They lead a life full of happiness and bliss.

The four contemplations are quite practical. In the context of preksha dhyana, we have accepted sixteen types of contemplation. Each contemplation is practised for months together and only then do they get assimilated into our lives. The practice of contemplation is an infallible solution for all problems and is the most divine step for reaching the pinnacle of spirituality.

ESSENCE

- A man can be truly spiritual only when he realizes the actual truth about materialism.
- Spirituality starts evolving when one realizes that his body and soul are separate.
- There is no happiness or sorrow associated with material objects when one realizes that they are actually separate from him.
- One whose consciousness of asharana is awakened realizes that the external material world does not provide any relief or shelter.
- When one realizes that his soul is separate from his body, he can easily overcome fear of suffering caused by disease, old age or death.
- A person who learns to live in solitude even in a crowd does not experience any kind of sorrow.

A person who has achieved spirituality through these four steps leads a pious and blissful life. Contemplation has to be practised for months together so that it can be assimilated into our lives. It is the best method for attaining spirituality.

15
JOY LIES WITHIN

The main motive behind men's various actions is to achieve freedom from misery and to experience joy. Imagination, expectations and actions have the same aim. Spirituality too aims at the same. Exerting oneself is meaningless if it does not result in such freedom. Nobody will have a motive to pursue it.

It has often been suggested that, to get rid of misery, we must do something other than merely closing our eyes and sitting in meditation. Why should we sit idle? Idleness will not help us procure the material objects without which we cannot get rid of misery. For those who entertain such thoughts, meditation is idleness. How can it free us from misery? Some philosophers believe that joy lies in attaining moksha, emancipation. What are the means of obtaining joy there? No body, no food, no meeting with friends; no thinking, no talking, nothing is there. What is the joy there? It appears to be a contradiction to say that we can get freedom from miseries through idleness or moksha.

UNDERSTANDING JOY AND SORROW

Material objects do give us some freedom from desire. Only food quenches hunger. Clothing can protect us from cold. A glass of cold water can satisfy a thirsty man. The shade of a tree gives relief to a person walking in the scorching heat. It is a reality that nobody can deny.

The question arises: What efforts are we making to get rid of hardships and wants? Religious people exhort us to practise religion in order to get freedom from misery. What does self-exertion provide us with? If it is incapable of fulfilling the needs of life, then, how can it relieve us from grief and misery? A spiritual practitioner is a destitute who owns neither property nor wealth. He does not exercise any authority or command, nor does he have any power.

These questions are raised by those who believe that only material objects are capable of giving us happiness. According to a spiritualist, however, material objects cannot give us true happiness. They may cure us of diseases but how can they give us happiness? For instance, we may eat to pacify our hunger but, does eating give us happiness? Not necessarily. Throughout our lives we eat something or the other to satisfy our hunger, but we confuse this with happiness. Eating something simply cures us of the pangs of hunger. A person who is addicted to intoxicants drinks when he becomes restless, and, for the time being, forgets his restlessness. But does the drink give him happiness? He's unaware of pain only as long as the intoxication lasts. Once the intoxication subsides, he will feel the pain again. What he gets is temporary relief from pain, he does not get happiness. Is music a source of joy? Music may not appeal to a sick person. Then how can we assume music to be a source of joy? A blanket which seems pleasing in winter is unwanted in summer. Are these material objects the real source of joy?

SPIRITUALISM: A ROAD TO HAPPINESS

Spiritualists have defined happiness as a process which starts in joy and ends in joy. Anything which gives relief for the time being but whose consequences are painful is not capable of giving joy. Joy is a continuous process which has no end. In other words, whatever gives us freedom from pain and whose consequences are also joyous is considered capable of giving happiness.

When soldiers win a battle, they are supposed to feel happy. Does their victory really result in happiness? It results only in grief and sorrow. The grief and sorrow are shared by the victors as well as by the vanquished ones. The devastation caused by war lasts for years and years. The after-effects of a war are most painful and unhappy. Let us try to understand this in order to find whether self-exertion is a source of joy.

Food increases as well as reduces pain. Food items are nutritive as well as harmful. According to Ayurveda, no food is completely nutritive or completely harmful. It is the quantity of food which is health-giving or harmful. For instance, arsenic can be a medicine as well as a poison, depending upon the amount we ingest. It is the quantity of medicine which produces harmful or agreeable consequences. Many things that we eat give temporary relief or pleasure. However, many of them are harmful in the long run. Ignorance in this matter results in a number of miseries. The pleasure obtained from the enjoyment of natural things often turns into pain. If this continues, our miseries will grow.

Some of us might feel that sadhana is a dry and unprofitable practice. This view is due to our attachment to material objects. The truth is that there can be no spiritual emancipation without going beyond the limitation imposed upon us by the material world. We are under the impression that bondage to material objects is a matter of joy. The general thinking in the modern world favours an increase in the production of material commodities, which can keep society happy and content. But the spiritualist believes that there can be no contentment or happiness without getting rid of this limitation. This creates two views—one which advocates the enjoyment of material objects and the other which advocates spiritual enjoyment.

The man of today, who suffers tension, is unable to appreciate the spiritual view; he advocates the enjoyment of material objects. Once he begins the practice of meditation, his tension begins to subside, the glandular secretion becomes balanced and the mind becomes calm. He can experience joy. His delusions disappear and his attachment to material objects reduces. The problem with the modern man is that, instead of taking full advantage of the spring of eternal joy within him, he runs after the perishable pleasures offered to him by the material world.

JOY LIES WITHIN

Once, an old woman was searching for a needle on the road outside her house. A few children playing there asked her what she was looking for. The woman replied that she had lost a needle in her room but as the room was utterly dark she thought it was advisable to search for it on the road. Acharya Bhikshu illustrated the same concept through a story. A man suffering from a visual disorder visited a physician, who gave him an ointment which he was advised to apply to his eyes. The patient returned home and applied the ointment to his back. On being asked, he replied, 'I am doing so because when I applied it to my eyes, there was a burning sensation. There is no such sensation when I apply it to my back.'

I would like to tell you another story. Once, a camel and an ox happened to live together. The camel was suffering from some disease and had to be stamped with an iron rod. A veterinarian came and, instead of stamping the camel, he stamped the ox. When he was asked why he had done so, he replied that his hand could not reach that part of the camel's body which was to be stamped and so he had stamped the ox instead. We can very well imagine the consequences of such foolishness.

It is difficult to imagine how many contradictory actions we do in our life. We laugh at others for such acts but, unconsciously, we do the same. The spring of joy lies within us but we search for it outside. We behave like the old woman. Sadhana puts an end to such foolish conduct. It makes us seek happiness within and stop searching for it in the material world.

We need two kinds of things: one kind which fulfils our material needs and the other which is capable of giving us joy and happiness. Spiritual exertion does not satisfy our material needs but does give us happiness and joy. Yet, we entertain delusions and confuse spiritual satisfaction with a total renunciation of worldly activities. If material objects were capable of giving us happiness, then modern man would have been the happiest creature in this world. The potential for production of material possessions has been raised sky-high and, yet, we are unhappy. The more material wealth we command, the unhappier we become. It is the wealthy who lose their peace of mind most easily, lose their sleep, sometimes even committing suicide. It is they who have to take tranquillizers to get sound sleep. Unlimited production and excessive consumption are the roots of our grief. We have to do some serious thinking on this subject. Industrially advanced countries tell us that they are capable of relieving us from misery, but even those countries have lost all sense of direction. They have gone astray and are groping in the dark. They themselves are in need of mental balance and peace.

The practitioner of sadhana is always alert. He labours to provide himself with the meaning of life. At the same time, he is aware of the fact that he has to avoid misery. He shields himself against the reactions to his actions, dissolves his delusions and attempts to obtain a clear vision. He is aware of what leads to misery and what gives him happiness. That is why he is capable of maintaining his mental equilibrium. Emotional imbalance is a special characteristic of the modern man. He is always perturbed. His experiences are continuously punctuated by sweetness as well as bitterness. Sometimes, they give him self-confidence, at other times he loses it. That is the result of mental imbalance.

Mental balance implies freedom from attachment and aversions; it also implies a sense of equality which is brought about by preksha. In it, the practitioner is full of delight as well as painful sensibility, but he tries to balance them. He tries to maintain and strengthen his equanimity. He aspires to be a pure spectator and to command pure knowledge.

ESSENCE

- The main motive behind spirituality is to achieve freedom from misery.
- Spiritualism, unlike material objects, gives permanent relief from pain.
- Joy is a continuous process, which material things are not capable of delivering.
- Sadhana requires one to go beyond the limitations of the material world.
- Due to our ignorance, we try to search outside for happiness, while the spring of joy is actually within us.
- Spiritualism does not satisfy material needs. But, if satisfying material needs were capable of making a man happy, this world would have been the happiest place to live in.
- The practitioner of sadhana maintains a mental equilibrium by avoiding attachments and aversions.
- Preksha dhyana helps achieve mental balance by strengthening equanimity.

16

EQUILIBRIUM: THE HIDDEN SECRET OF ABSOLUTE HAPPINESS

In *Uttaradhyana Sutra*, a prominent Jain canonical text, we find the description of absolute happiness. To be happy and to be absolutely happy are two different things. During a single day, how many times does a man shift between the states of joy and sorrow? We often notice that a person who had been happy a few minutes earlier becomes sad; there is a continuous fluctuation in man's moods. But one who has attained the state of absolute happiness will never become sorrowful.

The question arises here: what is the secret of absolute happiness? Equanimity in day-to-day life is the hidden secret of absolute happiness. The state of respect and disrespect, honour and dishonour keeps changing in a man's life. A person who knows the secret of spirituality can remain in any state. If we study the lives of great men, we will find that it is the quality of equilibrium that made them great. Defining the word yoga, the Gita says, 'Samatvam yoga muchyate' (equilibrium is yoga). At present, self-styled yogis have degraded its real meaning and purpose and turned it into a source of livelihood. The real meaning of yoga is practising equilibrium in daily life. One who remains balanced in every situation cannot be made sorrowful by anything. One who becomes happy on achieving honour or respect can also easily be made sorrowful by the slightest disrespect. Equilibrium is the secret of being free of transitory joy or sorrow.

Sorrow and imbalance are connected with each other. A man becomes sorrowful when he leads a life of imbalance. Acharya Bhikshu was a living example of a balanced life. Once, when he was on his way to a village, a man passing by asked, 'Who are you?' He replied, 'I am Bhikshu.' Hearing this, the man said disappointedly, 'Oh! What an inauspicious day! I will have to go to hell since I have seen your face in the morning.' Acharya Bhikshu asked, 'Oh! If this is true, then where will the person who sees your face in the morning go?' The man replied, 'To heaven, of course.' Acharya Bhikshu altered this answer into a positive situation and said, 'That is good for me, then. I will definitely go to heaven now.' This can only be the answer of a person who has mastered equilibrium.

The spiritual practice of equilibrium is the greatest path to achieving happiness. This practice does not include fasting or undertaking any difficulties. Only patience and self-realization are required. Great personalities like Sant Eknath, Dadu, Ramdas or Kabir did not have to undergo any training to acquire equilibrium. They all belonged to middle-class families and were not highly educated. But they immersed their minds in the search for the soul. They mastered the art of equilibrium and so, they remained uninfluenced by adverse circumstances.

UNDERSTANDING JOY AND SORROW

Equilibrium is the greatest achievement in the spiritual field. It is the way to constant happiness. Many people who visit me have a common complaint that they are unhappy. I experienced this especially during my visit to Punjab. I had always thought of Punjab as a very prosperous and happy state. But I was surprised to find that many people were unhappy. I advised them, 'Try to remain in balance. Don't get caught by the adverse situations.'

Once, there was a great king who had a loyal prime minister. The other ministers and courtiers were very jealous of him. They complained about the minister to the king who suspended him. Later, the king realized his mistake and reappointed him. He suspended the minister once again on some other grounds but reappointed him after realizing his mistake. This process went on and on. Some people asked the minister, 'Sir, you are suspended and reappointed, again and again. Don't you feel insulted? Why don't you approach the king? Don't you get irritated that you get suspended without being told the reason for your suspension?'

The minister said, 'I don't take anything to heart. When the king needs me, he appoints me and when he does not, he has the right to suspend me. When the king respects me, I consider it as respect to the position and when he insults me, I consider it as an insult to the position. So, there is no question of being angry. After all, it is the king's desire. Who am I to intervene in the king's desires?'

How can you make such a person sorrowful? A man who has learnt to live within himself, has made his thoughts positive, and has acquired a proper vision, cannot be disturbed, either by respect or by insult.

One who thinks only about the soul is able to awaken

EQUILIBRIUM: THE HIDDEN SECRET OF ABSOLUTE HAPPINESS

consciousness about equilibrium, while the one who thinks only about material things is unable to awaken it.

Once, a person visited a holy man and said, 'Oh holy one! Please teach me the art of equilibrium. My mind is very unsteady. Give me a lesson which will help me to proceed in the spiritual direction.' The holy man observed him carefully and said, 'Go and observe the idol outside the village.'

The person followed the holy man's orders and observed the idol. Many people passing by abused it. After a few days, the person returned to the holy man and said, 'I have been observing the idol during the last week. I do not understand why you asked me to do so.' The holy man asked him, 'What did you observe?' The person replied, 'The whole day, the people who passed by would abuse the idol and move on.' The holy man asked, 'Did the idol reply?' The person said, 'What could it say? It is merely a statue without any expression. It remains still.' The holy man then advised him, 'Behave like the idol. Don't get affected by what people say. That is the basis of the art of maintaining equilibrium. When you learn this, consider it the biggest lesson of spirituality.'

Unless and until we understand the secret of equilibrium, we will not be able to gain happiness.

Equilibrium in its highest form is attained by a veetraaga—one who is free of attachment and aversion. Only a veetraaga can attain eternal happiness. Other forms of happiness are momentary. The moods of the old, the youth and children keep on changing. What is the reason for such changes? The reason is that they are not searching for eternal happiness. If they searched for it, then, eventually, there would be no such fluctuations. With the end of such fluctuations, a person attains the happiness obtained from veetraagta—the state of being a veetraaga. The happiness felt by a veetraaga cannot be experienced by anyone else, not even the deities. Even Indra—the god of deities—cannot find that kind of happiness. The happiness of a veetraaga is incomparable. It is said in *Agamas*, the Jain scriptures, 'All the happiness of the world, when kept on one side of a balance, cannot outweigh the happiness achieved by veetraagas.'

Permanent happiness cannot be obtained without veetraagta. One who is not free of attachment, aversion, anger, pride and greed cannot achieve this kind of happiness. He will be happy one moment, and sad the next.

Once, a man, sitting in his office, was informed by his son, 'Our warehouse is on fire.' The man became upset. After some time, his second son informed him, 'Father, don't worry. Though our warehouse is on fire, the deal for the goods has already been completed.' The man became happy, thinking that the goods were not his any more to mourn the loss of. A little later, he was again informed by his son, 'There is bad news. The deal was completed but it had not been registered, so we have to bear the loss.' The man was disappointed once again. For the person who has not achieved veetraagta, happiness is only transitory.

To gain permanent happiness is really an arduous job. Lord Mahavira made many efforts to achieve it. He tolerated favourable and unfavourable situations. He never suffered from depression or frustration. Troubles never disturbed him. Why? It was because he was practising veetraagta. During that time, he realized that the soul and the body are separate. The body, not the soul, suffers pain. When the consciousness of veetraagta is awakened, troubles become trivial. Such a person never suffers from sorrow.

EQUILIBRIUM: THE HIDDEN SECRET OF ABSOLUTE HAPPINESS

There have been a number of great saints in Maharashtra, like Eknath, Namdev, Swami Ramdas, etc. They have attained the higher state in sadhana. Once, someone doubted Namdev's ability to control his anger and decided to test him. When Namdev was having his meal, the man came and sat on his shoulders. It would be normal for a person to get angry at such behaviour but Namdev said happily, 'I have a number of friends but you are the only dear friend who has sat so affectionately on my shoulders.' Only a person who has conquered anger can make such a statement.

The feelings of anger, hatred, fear and greed become an obstacle to achieving permanent happiness. There have been many inventions in the world—right from the needle to the atom bomb—but no invention has yet been made to produce happiness. The spiritual acharyas have discovered the secret of happiness and peace. They say, 'Walk on the path of veetraagta and you will always be happy.'

ESSENCE

- Equanimity in daily life is the hidden secret of absolute happiness.
- Sorrow and imbalanced thinking are connected with each other.
- A man with a materialistic outlook can never master the art of equilibrium.

MEDITATION: PERCEPTION OF THE BODY

1. **POSTURE:**
   Select a posture in which you can sit comfortably and continuously for forty-five minutes—full lotus, half lotus, cross-legged or diamond.

2. **MUDRAS—THE POSITION OF THE HANDS (ANY ONE):**
   i. Gyana Mudra:
      Place your right hand on the right knee and the left on the left knee, palms turned up. Touch the tip of the thumb with the tip of the index finger with a slight pressure. Keep the other fingers straight and relaxed.
   ii. Brahma Mudra:
      Place both hands on your lap, one above the other, palms turned up, the left palm under the right one. Keep your eyes softly closed.

3. **RECITATION OF MAHAPRANA DHVANI:**
   - Keep your lips softly closed, your spinal column and neck straight, without stiffness.
   - Inhale deeply and silently for about four to five

seconds, with a calm mind, empty of thoughts, all muscles relaxed.
- Concentrate on the top of your head.
- Keeping your lips closed, exhale slowly, making the sound of mmm ……… through the nostrils, like the buzzing of a bee.
- This may last eight to ten seconds. Inhale again and keep repeating this exercise for five minutes.

4. KAYOTSARGA (RELAXATION):
- Relax all the muscles in your body.
- Release all the stress from your body.
- Concentrate and allow your mind to travel, taking a trip to all the parts of your body, from the big toe of your right foot to the top of the head.
- Give an auto-suggestion to each and every muscle to relax and feel it relaxing.
- Concentrate deeply and remain completely alert.

5. PERCEPTION OF THE BODY

The practice consists of concentrating the mind on each part of the body, one by one, and perceiving the sensations and vibrations taking place in each part. Of course, here, the perception does not mean the visual perception, but the mental one. The sensations may be superficial sensations on the skin, such as the contact with the warmth or the coolness of your clothes, itching and perspiration, or they may be the sensations of pain, numbness, tingling, felt in the muscles, or the vibrations of the electrical impulses in the nervous system, or any other type of vibration. Starting from the surface, you have to penetrate deep inside, and try to become aware of the internal and subtle vibrations. Remain completely detached from the sensations; try to keep your mind free of likes and dislikes.

Concentrate your mind on the big toe of your right foot. Allow your concentration to spread and permeate throughout the entire toe. Perceive the sensations and vibrations taking place in that region. Become aware of them, experience them without any likes or dislikes; use deep concentration and remain fully alert.

Now, move your attention to each part of the right limb, one by one. I shall now name the part of your body on which you have to concentrate and perceive it: the other toes, the sole, the heel, the ankle, the upper part of the foot, the calf muscles, the knee, the thigh, up to the hip joint. Perceive the whole part, experience the sensations and vibrations taking place in each part. Maintain equanimity.

In the same way, practise the perception of all the parts of your left limb.

The trip of the lower body is now complete. Start the trip of the middle body from the waist up to the neck. Concentrate your mind on each part, one by one—perceive the waist, the navel, the abdomen including the

MEDITATION: PERCEPTION OF THE BODY

big intestine, the small intestine, the kidneys, the spleen, the liver, the pancreas, the duodenum, the stomach and the diaphragm. Then, the entire chest, including the lungs, the heart, the ribs, the throat and the vocal cords. Concentrate your mind and perceive.

Next, practise the perception of the entire portion of the back, including the spinal column, the spinal cord and the neck. Now concentrate on the entire portion of the right hand and arm, including the thumb, the fingers, the palm, the wrist, the lower arm, the elbow, the upper arm and the shoulder. Perceive each part, one by one. In the same way, concentrate on the left hand and arm. The trip of the middle body is complete.

Now, we come to the upper body. Concentrate your mind on each part, from the chin up to the head. The chin, the lips, the inside of the mouth—the tongue, the teeth, the palate; the cheeks, the nose; the right ear, all the three parts—the outer, the middle, and the inner; and the right temple. In the same way, the left ear and the left temple, the right eye, the left eye, the forehead and the head. Perceive each part, one by one. During the perception of the tongue, allow it to hang free, without touching any spot in the mouth.

While perceiving the head, perceive all the parts of your brain—the front, the back, the right, the left, the outer and the inner. Allow your mind to permeate throughout the brain. The trip of the upper body is complete.

UNDERSTANDING JOY AND SORROW

Now, practise the perception of the body as a whole. You may stand up slowly and carefully, keeping your eyes closed. Allow your mind to travel up from the big toes to the head and down from the head to the big toes rather quickly. Passing through each part of the body, perceive the vibrations within it. Experience the tingling sensation in each and every muscle, nerve, cell and the skin, produced by the contact of your conscious mind. You may also practise holding the breath, intermittently, for a while. Let yourself be completely absorbed in the perception of the body.

Lastly, allow your mind to travel through the body quite slowly. If you experience pain or any other peculiar sensation, you may stop there for a while and perceive it with equanimity, without any like or dislike.

Conclude the meditation session by chanting the mahaprana dhvani three times.

17

AMITY LEADS TO HAPPINESS

The key to happiness lies through amity. There are many facets of amity, as given below.

SOLITUDE AND AMITY

Solitude is one of the important aspects of spirituality. Those who have learnt to live in solitude can establish harmony with the present moment. Now the question arises: why then is amity given equal importance to spirituality? The answer needs to be searched within.

Man keeps seeking truth with the help of spirituality and science. But they both serve different purposes. The truth being searched for by science is only to develop physical and material comforts. The result of such developments has been quite discouraging and destructive. It has created a negative impact on social, moral and ethical fronts, giving rise to fear, enmity and brutality.

The aim of searching for the truth through spirituality is to strengthen amity. 'Seek truth within and have amity with all'—is an important message of spirituality. It is a universal axiom that he who has cultivated the virtue of amity can also master the art of living in solitariness. The search for truth that does not culminate in amity is no longer beneficial to humanity. Amity comes as a beautiful boon to human life. Those who nourish it live a prosperous and healthy life.

HEALTH AND AMITY

Medical science may say that germs are the cause of various diseases. But, it has been found that as soon as emotions of hostility crop up, the morale gets weakened. This reduces the body's power for resistance. Any increase in the feeling of enmity will lead to deterioration in a man's health.

A person who has not developed amity has a weak morale. Enmity is like a poison which harms whomsoever it strikes. It weakens the morale, creates disappointment, and increases hatred. Hatred, depression, jealousy, greed are the vicious germs that keep on spoiling health and making life miserable.

The first and foremost benefit of amity is good health. Everyone wants to be healthy. It has been proved that those who are filled with friendly inclinations have good immunity and remain healthy. When a person falls sick, he takes medicines; in alternative therapies, he takes shelter in remedies like yoga, Ayurveda, etc. Spirituality provides shelter, while medicine is an aid for good health. Shelter and aid are quite different. Though aid can be taken temporarily, one needs to find a permanent shelter, and that is to be found in spirituality. One who seeks shelter in medicines is apt to lose his health, but he who finds shelter in spirituality protects himself and develops physical harmony.

Jayacharya wrote a book titled *Aradhana*, in which he described the beauty of feeling comfortable with sickness.

'When sickness crops up, I should endure it with affection and hold it lovingly, instead of opposing and fighting it.' If not, you will experience deep mental agony. Today's psychologists are confident that they will be able to evolve a psychic conduct which would guide the patient so that he learns to tolerate pain without the support of medicines.

Our physical system has an inbuilt capacity to tolerate a lot of pain. It can form substances to lessen the pain. But when one's mental strength subdues the pain, it is an attempt to be friendly with the ailment. Our mental make-up should be designed to liberate us from fear, worry and tension.

Man gets tense and drowns himself in a ocean of worries and, consequently, aggravates his pain by 5 to 50 per cent. If we develop fearlessness and become tension-free, then, we will not feel even 5 per cent of the 50 per cent pain which we are suffering. Pain is not experienced equally by all; nor does a person always experience pain in the same way because fear and worry exacerbate the pain. Some people are cowards and literally cry over trifles. Others are fearless to the extent that they do not cry over a molehill. Actually, our mental and emotional conditions are instrumental to the presence or absence of pain.

To grow in fearlessness is to establish amity with sickness and pain. To become free of tension and suffering is to establish an amicable relationship with the ailment. We see people suffering badly, but their strength lies in centring their faith in disease, and the pain gets relieved. Faith is important for establishing amity with pain. Man changes tremendously with the transformation of his feelings. The sooner the emotions are transformed, the sooner man changes. We do not realize that, with the transformation of feelings, our body chemicals, too, change.

INNER BEAUTY AND AMITY

Only those who have a deep desire to establish amity can realize true happiness. Many people get angry and upset at the mere sight of some persons. This will continue till they develop the virtue of amity towards everybody. The sight of a child sitting and playing makes a captivating and fascinating picture. Its peace and beauty is due to magnanimous waves and pure feelings. A person who exhibits friendly behaviour automatically becomes beautiful regardless of his outer appearance. Mahatma Gandhi was not physically attractive, but a Western thinker described him as the most beautiful person. His personality and conduct revealed a tremendous inbuilt capacity for amity.

HAPPINESS AND AMITY

Eternal and stable happiness comes as a boon of amity. A person who has developed this quality will never be sad. When amity is not cultivated, a person tends to develop feelings of hatred. A person who has built up amity never gets provoked by anyone or by any act.

Jesus Christ once decided to visit the house of a prostitute in order to preach to her. His disciples questioned him, 'Lord, where are you going?' Jesus replied, 'I am going where I am supposed to go.' His disciples were baffled and said, 'She is unchaste and non-religious. You should not go there.' Jesus replied, 'Therefore I must go there.' Jesus visited the prostitute's house. His disciples and devotees felt hatred and aversion towards her, but Jesus had no such feelings. Where there is harmony, there is no place for hostility. We should hate the evil and not the evildoer. Mahatma Gandhi used to say, 'Hate the sin, not the sinner.'

HUMOUR AND AMITY

Friendly emotions developed through amity acquire a sense of humour. Humour is like a flower that spreads its fragrance and beauty around. It is difficult for everyone to be humorous; this quality can only be achieved through amity.

Acharyashree Tulsi had a good sense of humour. Once, a person who advocated a conflicting philosophy came to Acharyashree. He questioned him, 'Sir, my son has disappeared. Should I search for him? If I do, will it be a sacred act or a sin?' Acharyashree understood and replied cleverly, 'Your question is very strange. You did not ask for my advice when you planned to have a son. You did not question then whether it was a sacred act or a sinful one. Now, when wondering whether to search for him, you are bothered whether it would breed sin or not. The answer to your question would be the same in both the cases.' The visitor got the message and went away silently.

A person filled with amity can develop a sense of humour. Those who wish to develop feelings of amity have to struggle a lot. Hostility requires no struggle. If a person who is willing to pursue the sadhana of friendliness does not develop a sense of humour, he is quite likely to break down while facing problems.

It is true that only a person with humour can sustain and survive on the difficult path of disappointments and rejections. Humour is the outcome of friendliness. That is why the important objective of spirituality is to search for truth and to develop friendliness.

BIOELECTRICITY AND AMITY

Bioelectricity is still a mystery for most of us although our life is governed by it. It is the subtlest and most powerful force determining our life and its conditions. Enmity weakens bioelectricity and gradually destroys it. People with weak bioelectricity have neither immunity nor joy in their lives. Happiness is nothing but powerful bioelectricity.

The feeling of amity increases the bioelectricity in our lives. It strengthens our vital energy. That is why when someone practises preksha dhyana, he understands the power of meditation, and he will definitely stress upon the power of bioelectricity and its development through amity.

The development of amity will pave the way for the development of health, happiness, bioelectricity and peace. For these benefits, one must cultivate amity. And for their development, one must practise preksha dhyana. Participation in a ten-day camp will help you realize your inner self and develop amity.

ESSENCE

- Learning to live in solitude helps develop amity.
- Amity increases immunity while hostility weakens the body's ability to resist.
- Advantages of amity:
  - Helps maintain good health.
  - Increases inner beauty.
  - Happiness comes as a by-product of amity.
  - Humour developed with amity helps one walk on the difficult path of rejections and disappointments.
  - Increases the bioelectricity in our lives and strengthens vital energy.

18
STANDING ALONE IN A CROWD

Society is full of contradictory forces which continuously produce conflicts which, again, draw a man towards sorrow. Man has an independent existence but he has to adjust with all these forces and live in society. The only way to be free of such conflicts is to experience solitude even in a crowd.

LIVING ALONE

The journey of spirituality lies in enjoying solitariness. Lord Mahavira prescribed a number of sutras for spiritual practice. To isolate oneself in a solitary place is one of them. That is the highest achievement of anyone's life. A person who masters the art of enjoying solitariness is fortunate. Living alone is difficult and, generally, a man is scared of it. He feels insecure and so he always desires company.

Someone once remarked, 'The birth rate of twins is increasing these days.' The other person asked him, 'So, why does that surprise you?' He said, 'The incidence of violence, crime, etc. is growing day by day. That makes a child so insecure that he prefers to come along with a partner.' This is one of the saddest comments on the present times. It seems that today's world is filled with fears. Thus, although solitariness leads to spiritual achievement, loneliness creates fear.

SOLITUDE: AN ANSWER TO THE SEARCH FOR TRUE JOY

A man wants peace, bliss, energy, and he tries to search truth for them. Where can a man find all these virtues? Do they lie in this world or will they be found in some other world? Actually, they are all present in our own environment. We are surrounded by peace. Every nook and corner is replete with truth. An incessant stream of bliss is flowing around us. We are surrounded by these virtues but they are not witnessed by us. The reason for this is our careless attitude towards them. We never try to search for true joy around us. We pretend to have a busy lifestyle.

A busy person cannot stay alone. And a man who knows how to live in solitariness will never suffer from lack of time or the burden of a busy lifestyle. Practice of solitariness requires meditation. But, if a person is asked to do meditation or some other spiritual practice, then, he generally finds an excuse pleading lack of time. Everyone gets twenty-four hours in one day, but those who do not know how to manage time will always remain busy; they will never find the time.

A child was studying in his room. There was a power cut, but the child still continued. His father came up and asked, 'What are you doing?' He replied, 'I am studying.' The father, surprised, asked, 'How can you study in this darkness?' The child said, 'I was so engrossed in my studies that I didn't realize that there was a power cut.' He was merely pretending to be busy and, in reality, his actual purpose was not being served.

It is a big error to conceal one's mistakes. One who remains continuously occupied cannot experience solitariness, and one who does not experience solitariness cannot realize truth. There are twelve contemplations in Jain yoga, of which the contemplation of solitariness is one. It means to experience solitariness while living in a social world. One who is unaware of the concept of solitariness cannot save himself from unfavourable situations and undesirable behaviour.

SOLITUDE IN SOCIETY

Undesirable situations are created because a man considers all his relationships as reality. Relationships are temporary connections between individuals. We build relationships for our own convenience. And when we start considering these temporary relationships as permanent, they become a cause for sorrow. A person gets angry when something according to his will is not carried out. That happens because he forgets the individuality of others. If he always keeps this fact in mind, he will respect the importance of others for the same reasons. 'If I have the right to take independent decisions, then others, too, have that right.' If he keeps to this right vision, he can lead a smooth social life.

If society is important, then, every individual in it is of greater importance. We have organized society for our own convenience and utility. But, when prime importance is given to society and an individual is treated as secondary, problems arise. Only those social systems in which an individual is given adequate importance have remained successful.

Sometimes, to obtain certain results, one thing is given primary importance and others are treated as secondary. When we walk, we put one foot forward, leaving the other behind.

But, with the next step, the foot that has been left behind comes forward. Only then does motion become possible, not if we prevent the other foot from coming forward. But, in the present times, we are not following this practice. We concentrate on society, ignoring the individuals who form it. We put obstacles in the way of our own progress, making the life of individuals unhappy. This, in turn, has made our own lives unhappy.

A son deceives his father, a husband deceives his wife and, similarly, a wife may cheat on her husband. A person who knows the importance of individual existence and the art of enjoying solitariness will never be saddened by such incidents, but will accept them as part of human nature. He will never be burdened with sorrow. On the other hand, a man who is ignorant of the importance of solitariness will indulge in sorrow over the deceit for years. The fact that a dear one has deceived him makes the incident unforgettable. It keeps on haunting him, making his life miserable.

There was a king during Lord Mahavira's time. He was totally detached from all kinds of worldly pleasures. He wanted to search for eternal joy so he decided to take diksha—the act of renouncing the world. He did not want his son to be his successor either. There was no ill feeling behind this decision but he did not want him to get involved in the violence and other vicious acts attached to ruling over a kingdom, thinking that it would be an obstacle to his spiritual life. Keeping this idea in his mind, he entrusted his kingdom to his nephew. The prince, unaware of his father's thoughts, was filled with a feeling of revenge. He thought, 'My father is my biggest enemy. No father in the world can be as inconsiderate as mine.' He was filled with these ill feelings and wanted to retaliate. His father had become a holy man, and his cousin, the king. He began to live a miserable life, preoccupied with ill will. The minister came to know about the prince's mental condition and tried to console him. He made him understand the importance of religion and amity. The prince was religious and, being a Jain, he used to celebrate the festival of forgiveness—kshamapana divas. On this occasion, it is customary to repent one's intentional as well as unintentional wrong behaviour and deeds towards everybody in the world. The prince declared, 'I apologize to everyone except my father'. With the feelings of revenge within, he could never live the rest of his life in peace.

Let us try to understand the human psychology involved in taking decisions, keeping relationships in mind. The prince accepted relationships as everything. But, according to the spiritual point of view, a man should never think that relations and individuals are separate.

'Experience solitariness while living in society' is one of the most important aphorisms for transforming consciousness. One needs to keep a balance between individual and society. A person who practises spirituality will always keep in mind: 'I am alone and my relationship with society is temporary. All these contacts, all these relations, all these social systems and orders—I accept them, I live them, I follow them but, ultimately, I am an independent individual.' No external circumstances can make such a man unhappy.

Gurdjieff, a famous Russian spiritual teacher, developed a spiritual exercise based on this aphorism. In this exercise, twenty to thirty people stayed together in a hall for three months. They carried out their daily activities in solitariness, contemplating, 'I am alone.' This practice is similar to the one explained in ancient Jain scriptures. It proves that the truth of solitariness is universal, irrespective of time and place. A person living anywhere in the world will have to practise this aphorism if he wants to experience universal happiness.

SOLITARINESS AND THE INDIVIDUAL

There are three progressive stages of solitariness:
- Practising living alone
- Experiencing solitariness everywhere
- Walking alone in a crowd

Today, it has become a fashion to imitate others for material pleasure. People do not think whether the imitation is morally right or not. A man lies, cheats and exploits others. If he is questioned, his reply will most probably be, 'Everyone does it. Why should I not?' At present, everyone thinks the same way.

We look at society from this point of view: we think that everybody does it and if we don't—will it make a difference? If nobody acts honestly, our doing otherwise will make no difference. These considerations take us away from truth. One who realizes solitariness will never argue about what everybody in society is doing. His viewpoint will always be, 'What am I doing?' and not what others are doing. He will think about his duty from the moral point of view before taking any action. This thinking dawns only with the realization of solitariness. It gives us the strength to walk alone on the righteous path.

A Sanskrit poet has written, 'A bee can bore into wood and come out of it but it cannot escape from a closed lotus.' Here, the bondage of attachment makes the lotus petals stronger than wood. This bondage of false and transitory attachment is the biggest hindrance in the realization of solitariness. Attachment brings the greatest sorrow.

The first lesson to be learnt in order to practise solitariness is to break the bondage of attachment. We should never forget the eternal truth of solitariness. Initially, it may sound unreal and harsh but, with the realization of truth, one can rest in peace and secure oneself from all types of sorrow. 'Walk alone' is a powerful aphorism for increasing self-esteem. It does not mean one should cut off oneself totally from society or relationships, but that one should always remember and realize the eternal truth, 'I exist alone.' Once this art is mastered, one can face any kind of adversity and make one's life happy.

ESSENCE

- The journey to spirituality starts with learning to enjoy solitariness. Living in solitude is one of the highest achievements on the spiritual front.
- We are surrounded by joy, bliss, peace and other virtues but we cannot experience them because we are too busy.
- One who is continuously occupied cannot be in solitude and, hence, cannot experience truth and save himself in unfavourable situations.
- Man considers relationships to be permanent; he forgets his own as well as others' individuality, thereby laying the ground for undesirable situations.
- A society which is treated as being more important than the individuals that form it cannot flourish for a long time.
- A person who practises solitude even in society, thinking, 'I exist alone', is never burdened with sorrow.
- Solitude is truly regardless of time and place.
- For an individual, the progressive steps to solitariness include practising living alone, experiencing solitariness around himself, and finally, having the capacity to practise it even in a crowd.
- The thoughtless imitation of immoral acts is prevalent. One can only think about morality if one practises solitariness.
- To achieve solitariness, one needs to break the bondage of attachment and practise the aphorism, 'Walk alone.'

19

HAPPINESS THROUGH DETACHMENT

The senses are the means and the sources of joy as well as of sorrow. A source that is common to both can never be said to be a source of eternal happiness. Senses are meant to perform their respective functions of perception. The existence of senses is not a problem in itself. Eyes are meant for seeing and seeing is not the problem. The problem arises only when we attach ourselves to the object seen and forget everything else. Attachment is not through the senses; they are only the means. Those who move in the world of senses and yet are successful in keeping the senses in harmony, free of attractions and aversions, will find peace and tranquillity.

Ravishanker was a famous holy man of Gujarat. He spent his life in public service. A man said to him, 'Sir, I am not able to give up alcohol.' The holy man asked, 'Brother, why can't you give up alcohol?' The man explained, 'The alcohol has caught hold of me so strongly that I cannot give it up. Please give me some remedy.' Ravishanker said, 'Come after three or four days, I shall tell you the remedy then.'

The man returned after four days. He found Ravishanker holding a pillar. The man said, 'Please come, I want to speak to you.' The holy man said, 'I cannot come. The pillar is holding me.' The other man asked, 'Sir, how can the pillar hold you?' Ravishanker repeated, 'I am quite sure that I cannot come.' The man asked, 'Sir, can you not understand the simple fact that you are holding the pillar, the pillar is not holding you.' The holy man retorted, 'You are right!' The man said, 'If you let go, you will be relieved of the pillar.' Ravishanker immediately spread out his arms and was free. Then he said, 'Is it applicable only to me or to you too? You have caught hold of the alcohol, it has not caught hold of you.' The man understood the truth. What attaches you to another object exists only within you. The object does not hold the man, the man holds the object. This is known as attachment. There is an entity within man which keeps getting attached to everything, holding on to everything. Whatever comes, it holds on to that.

The senses are simply the means; they are not at all responsible for attachment. As regards colour, sound and taste, the eyes, ears and tongue are meant to perceive things as they are. That is their job. The entity within us is responsible for causing attachment. We have to seek the methodology which will teach us to treat objects as objects only, and which will prevent us from getting attached to them. Is it possible for us to take objects as objects only and nothing else? Yes, it is. We should not get swayed by like and dislike for the objects and thereby, land ourselves in a vicious circle of attachment.

Attachment is very active and effective. As soon as you put something on your tongue, you say, 'Oh! How tasty this is!' Or,

'How tasteless this is!' Both the tastes are wedded to it. The matter, in itself, is neither tasty nor without taste, then, why are adjectives like tasty and tasteless, good and bad associated with it? That is because something exists within us that segregates things into good and bad, ugly and beautiful. We can enter into a new world only after we get to know the entity within us which causes us to form an attachment to worldly objects and propensities. As long as we are unaware of it and are unable make it ineffective, we cannot be free from the world of likes and dislikes, that is, the world of senses. When matter is treated as only matter, then, that world is known as 'the world beyond the senses'. The man existing in this sensual world can never solve his problems. He is always entangled in the duality of the likes and dislikes of this world. Because of this perpetual bewilderment, he never gets liberation. Thus, his happiness is utterly transitory and fleeting. Today, if the food is tasty, he is pleased and he praises it. Tomorrow, if the food is not to his taste, then he will be enraged because he is deprived of tasty food. The problem can be solved through the practice of detachment.

Attachment can be transformed into detachment and asceticism can be developed. Psychology recognizes that man has some basic mental tendencies. There are approximately fourteen mental tendencies, such as those for feeling hungry, thirsty, lustful, for quarrelling, etc. In the world of philosophy, man has the impression of action, in the form of karmic imprints bounded by the actions done in the previous births. In the world of psychology, we are bound by basic mental propensities and, in the world of philosophy, we are compelled by the result of our previous actions. Attachment works through us and we are slaves to it, according to both the streams. Then, how can we think of a change? How do we change man, society, our beliefs and our lifestyles?

The doctrine of karma states that the results of karma can be changed. Psychologists say that basic mental inclinations can be purified. This can happen if one experiences one's existence separate from the body and the senses. This can be done only through meditation.

Meditation does not directly change a habit. It only appears to us as if the habit has been changed due to meditation. It would be a frivolous gain if it were only mediation that changed the habit. If the habit is changed but the cause still remains dormant, it will crop up again, like the budding of trees in spring. We have to change the causal element which nourishes the habit. We have to dive deep within ourselves. In preksha dhyana camps, participants are taught to perceive the body from within. The body is merely the medium, we have to actually perceive within. We should learn to seek and look inside, our mind should not always be wandering outside. We should not focus merely on the external body. The body is a combination of bones, blood, flesh, etc. Then, what do we seek within the body? In body awareness, we perceive bones, flesh, blood, marrow, the nervous system and the endocrine system, but we also have to perceive something else within. In fact, we have to perceive the one entity that is driving our habits, getting the work done by us. That driving force is the vibration and the sensation inside the body. We have several vibrations which work through us. We have to perceive these vibrations or waves which are active and regulate our activities. If a person tells a lie, it is these waves which are acting behind it. If someone commits a theft, it is the negative movement of the waves behind that theft. A man commits a murder because the waves guide him. The waves existing in our body can be compared to the waves existing in an ocean. Our body is also like the ocean.

Medical science has observed that 80 per cent of the body consists of water. The body attempts to perceive those sensations and vibrations which drive our tendencies. That is a biochemical reaction which generates different types of chemicals. Those chemicals are responsible for several changes and results. We have to perceive the vibrations and realize each vibration of the body separately, feel it deep within us. We have to understand the subtlety and the essence of holding each vibration distinctly, and then we can definitely transcend the senses and attain the condition of non-attachment. The transformation of sensual objects is possible only when we are able to hold the vibrations. Why should I do this job? The job is being driven by the vibrations. Why should I obey the vibrations? Then only will detachment come. When we grasp the play of senses and understand that we should not become a slave to them, only then will detachment mature. This is not an impossible task.

A man came to a holy person and said, 'I want to do sadhana. Please direct me to a guru.' The holy man said, 'Go to the king of this town. You will learn sadhana from him.' The man said, 'Why should I go to the king? If the king knew sadhana then why did you become a holy man?' The holy man said, 'Do not argue unnecessarily. Go to the king.' He went to the king, who was engrossed in the affairs of his kingdom. He told the king, 'The holy man has directed me to you, kindly give me the knowledge of sadhana.' The king told him to sit down. He waited the whole day. He saw that the king was busy in his activities throughout the day, taking care of the administration.

When the affairs of the kingdom had been dealt with, the king said, 'Come, let's take a bath.' He went with the king and wondered why the holy man had directed him to the king. What kind of sadhana could he learn? As there was no alternative, he followed the king. A river was flowing behind the palace. Both of them stepped into it. Suddenly, they noticed that the king's palace had caught fire. He further observed that the king was unmoved. He told the king that his palace was engulfed by fire. The king responded, 'That is not my problem!'

Though the king was relaxed, the man ran to the palace in which he had left his bag. He brought it and informed the king that the fire was increasing. The king remained undisturbed. Eventually, the fire was extinguished. The man asked the king, 'Oh king! Why did you not pay attention to the fire?' The king said, 'Earlier, I used to worry, but now, I have transcended my likes and dislikes, and have become free of sensations and vibrations. A palace is only a place to dwell in. I am entirely separate from it. I am not the palace nor am I attached to it. In the true sense, it is not mine. Then why should I be bothered whether it burns down or collapses?' The man grasped the essence of sadhana—he was attached to his bag and had run to save it, while the king, being detached, remained calm and unworried, witnessing the greedy fire engulfing his palace. That was how the man learnt the essence of sadhana from the king.

The important doctrine of preksha dhyana is to destroy the thread of likes and dislikes. For this, we have to delve deep within us and hold those vibrations which emerge from the subtlest body, and diffuse them. The process of preksha dhyana is the methodology of cutting the thread of sensations and vibrations. We should cultivate this practice in order to cultivate the capacity to change ourselves.

ESSENCE

- The problem arises only when we attach ourselves to the object seen and forget everything else.
- The senses are simply the means, they are not at all responsible for attachment.
- When matter is treated as only matter, then that world is known as 'the world beyond the senses'.
- Mental inclinations and imprints can be purified when a man experiences his existence as separate from his physical body.

20

ACHIEVING HAPPINESS BY GOING BEYOND THE MIND

~

Once, Maharshi Patanjali was asked a question: 'How can a person achieve happiness?'

He said, 'Nirvichar vaishaardya atmaprasaad.' (Going beyond thoughts paves the way to spirituality and, thereby, happiness can be obtained.)

There are some obstacles which prevent us from going beyond thoughts. Until these obstacles are removed, happiness cannot be achieved.

A holy man was pleased with one of his disciples who served him well. He decided to give him something. He called the disciple and gave him a stone covered with a cloth which was attached to a pair of tongs. He said, 'This is parasmani, the philosopher's stone which can turn iron into gold by mere touch. Be prosperous and live happily.'

The disciple was doubtful about the ability of the stone and **touched it with a needle.** It immediately turned into gold. Still, he doubted the stone and asked the holy man, 'Are you making a fool of me?'

The holy man was surprised and said, 'Why do you ask that? You saw that the needle turned into gold. Where then is the question of doubting it?'

The disciple said, 'The stone was tied to the iron tongs, then, why didn't they turn to gold?'

The holy man said, 'Your doubt is appropriate. But there was a layer of cloth between the stone and the tongs. So they did not come into direct contact with each other.'

The disciple was now free of doubt. In the same way, the source of happiness lies within. Happiness is the inborn quality of consciousness. This happiness can be exposed outside but there are some impediments which stop its flow.

We can attain constant happiness only after we have abandoned the activities of the mind. As long as the mind is active, one cannot attain constant happiness. It acts as a barrier, like the cloth. Thinking acts as a big hindrance. The mind goes on moving, from one word, one idea, one process, to another. It remains active even when it is being concentrated. The activities of the mind are so subtle that they mislead us into believing that we have ceased to think. The fact is that, in the state of concentration, the mind is active with reference to a single subject only. It only lessens the fickleness of the mind, a temporary absence of jumbled-up mental activities. One cannot think about other subjects and concentrate at the same time. The two cannot go together.

'NIRVICHAR DHYANA' MEDITATION

We can attain nirvichar dhyana, a state where one goes 'beyond thoughts'. Nirvichar meditation means nurturing the mind into a natural state of pure consciousness. It implies pure knowledge and nothing else. Nirvichar means clear and clean knowledge. It is pure comprehension or direct perception. In this sense, one can attain keval gyana, complete knowledge, even today. We should not think that the age of keval gyanis—those who attain keval gyana—is over. If people could attain keval gyana in the past, there is no reason why we may not attain it today. As soon as the mind stops wandering, and it has merged into the soul, mental activities come to be replaced by spiritual activities. Keval gyana is not intellectual but spiritual knowledge.

KEVAL GYANA

The word 'keval' has two meanings—pure and perfect. When knowledge is accompanied by samvedana (feelings), it is neither pure nor perfect. It becomes pure only when it is free of all feelings. Pure knowledge is the activity of the soul. When the soul is free of feelings it begins to shine like pure light. It becomes perfect. The state of nirvichar is a state of upayoga which means the innate activity of the soul or consciousness. In such a state, all feelings and sensations cease.

CONCENTRATION

The first step to attaining the state of nirvichar is concentration. It is a form of training the mind. Fickleness is a natural tendency of the mind, which always remains scattered and which never sticks to a single point. A stable mind seems more or less an unnatural entity. It is often compared to mercury which cannot be arrested. In the same way, it is assumed that one cannot arrest the mental processes. People have been wondering for thousands of years how to arrest these mental processes. Man is an ingenious being and has devised methods of forming small balls of mercury. In the same way, with the help of meditation, he can arrest the fleeting mental process also.

Concentration fixes the mind on a definite point. This releases enormous mental energy. But concentration needs a lot of exertion. It is difficult to make the mind concentrate even for a few hours. An hour's concentration uses up a lot of energy.

Concentration of the mind is the first step in meditation and, eventually, meditation leads us to permanent happiness. We have to concentrate the mind on a single subject or thought. In this state, the mental process begins to flow in one direction only. The stage of concentration should not be considered the final stage. What we perceive in the state of concentration is only a modification of the mind. We see objects and we hear sounds which have nothing to do with concentration. The state of concentration is not the state of self-perception.

Constant happiness demands pure consciousness. Consciousness which is occupied by false notions generates pain and trouble. In a state of pure consciousness, one does not make a distinction between happiness and misery, good and bad, friends and foes, life and death. All are one and the same thing in the state of equanimity. Yoga is the state of equanimity which is the culmination of spiritual exertion, and which is free of all kinds of miseries.

REALIZING THE SOUL BY NIRVICHAR

But the soul, the core of our existence, can be realized only in the state of nirvichar. It seems odd to think that there exists something which cannot be realized by our mind or realized through thinking. Words, ideas and thoughts are not the media through which one can arrive at the self. It is impossible to imagine through the normal mental process what the soul is.

A complete halt to these mental processes is the pre-condition for self-realization. It is an essential message of the scriptures. The normal experiences of life are based on knowledge and the various kinds of feelings associated with it. We cannot then think what is beyond them. Our limitations do not allow us to think that there may be things other than those which we come across through the medium of the senses and the mind.

The life we live is based on sensory experiences and mental processes which, by their very nature, are fleeting and temporary. But there are moments when we begin to feel that there may be something beyond sense experiences and the mind. Joy is the native characteristic of the self and it can be achieved by complete isolation of the self from the world of common experiences. The state of self is an autonomous state. It is the state of undifferentiated and undivided consciousness. In the ordinary experiences of life, consciousness remains split up into separate individual experiences.

We have to collect these individual experiences so that they may begin to flow in a single, undivided current like a mighty river. Concentration and meditation are the means of collecting the life force so that it may cease to flow in different directions. The mind, sense organs, thoughts and imagination keep the soul wandering here and there. They divide the self, as it were. They keep the life force weak and ineffective.

Once the flow of the self becomes centralized, it gains strength. It is an extrasensory and extra-mental state in which the soul becomes powerful, and manifests its characteristic joy. In order to achieve this state of the self, we have to come out of the mental processes and enter into a state of nirvichar. We have to watch and control the activities of the mind very carefully so they do not lead us astray. In other words, we have

ACHIEVING HAPPINESS BY GOING BEYOND THE MIND

to keep watch on ourselves. We have been given to believe that the age through which we are passing is not favourable to self-realization, with the result that we have lost all initiative and have become mechanical. However, life does not stand still. We must move forward. A man who watches over himself will deliberately move forward and towards a consciously characterized personality.

Thus, the state of constant happiness and self-consciousness can be attained only after we have abandoned the mind and reached the state of nirvichar. The exercise of the 'perception of breathing' in preksha dhyana is a way of attaining it. In it, a person initially concentrates on the breathing and, later, it helps him to dive deep inside. Through experience and by perceiving the inhalation and exhalation, gradually, we shall progress to a state where we will feel free of all thoughts and thereby achieve the state of nirvichar.

ESSENCE

- Going beyond thoughts paves the way to spirituality.
- We can attain real happiness only after we have abandoned the activities of the mind.
- Nirvichar meditation means nurturing the mind into a natural state of pure consciousness.
- A man who watches over himself will deliberately move forward towards a consciously characterized personality.

# 21

HAPPINESS AND FEARLESSNESS

Happiness is the greatest achievement of joy and sorrow. Each man passes through joy and sorrow. Joy is no great thing because, behind every joy, there lurks some sorrow. Sorrow, likewise, is not completely bad because it is invariably followed by joy.

Happiness lies beyond joy and sorrow. It virtually signifies purity of the mind. A mind that is pure is not ruffled by joy or sorrow. Happiness is like the pure sky, where there are no clouds, no rain, no hurricane—there is absolutely nothing. The sky is perfectly clear. Happiness is the condition of an unsullied mind. There are, however, many hurdles and dangers to be crossed before one can achieve such happiness. But even a major accomplishment, if attained without effort, loses something of its status, and is consequently ranked as minor. How many valleys have been crossed? How many ups and downs have been scaled? These are the questions posed while assessing a great achievement. The destination arrived at when the feet, tired of walking, come to the breaking point, becomes more significant and memorable.

Happiness is a tremendous achievement. Happiness and complete absence of fear go together. They are inseparably linked to each other. Where there is a total absence of fear, happiness is bound to be, and where there is happiness, fearlessness is its inevitable accompaniment. As soon as fear appears, happiness dissolves.

Man's life is tied to the wheel of circumstances. It is an interminable series without any break. There are seven circumstances which destroy happiness and create fear. It is essential to know them:
- Fear of this world;
- Fear of the other world;
- Fear of likes and dislikes;
- Sudden fear;
- Fear of suffering;
- Fear of death;
- Fear of disgrace.

THE COUNTENANCE OF FEAR

Thinking born out of fear is negative and destructive. A fearful man is incapable of thinking right; fear dulls his mind and heart; his thinking becomes blunt. It is futile to expect a fear-ridden brain to function normally. Such a brain cannot think constructively. The first condition for sane thinking is total freedom from fear. The mind, the brain and, indeed, the whole environment, should be free from fear. Only in the right atmosphere will sane thinking become possible.

Why are we afraid? Why is man ridden by fear? Fear is the outcome of wrong thinking. A man's individuality is determined by his thoughts. He has accepted certain ideas and beliefs, and his aura is vitiated by fear. A man who has understood even a little bit of spirituality, whose dry and anguished existence has been ever so lightly touched by the grace of religion, cannot but be fearless. He who is not fearless cannot be spiritual or religious, he cannot be sane. Fear is the root of all diseases, of all conflicts and of all non-spirituality. Can a fearful man experience truth? People talk endlessly of the soul and of God, but they live in delusion. How can a man, ridden by fear, know anything of highly subtle and supra-sensual elements? The mind is never free from fear—fear of health, fear of old age, fear of death and separation, fear of loss of people and things. The mind is ever dominated by fear, the power of consciousness is quite overthrown thereby, and one talks of the soul and of God. Will the soul manifest itself in a state of fear? Never. Fear can only give birth to a goblin; it cannot lead us to the soul or to God. Fear is the creator of evil spirits; for many people, it takes the form of a ghost or a demon. It is a kind of mental projection: in the very moment of fear, a ghost begins to take shape before our eyes; it is the projection, the idol, the reaction of a fear-afflicted mind. Is such a mind capable of any subtle penetration?

Fear is inevitably linked with the body-perception, which has two aspects—perception of the body and perception of something that is beyond the physical organism. He who perceives only the body creates more fear; the mere perception of the body is the root of all fear. The man whose vision does not go beyond the body will never know true fearlessness.

All unconsciousness proceeds from the body, and the unawareness of this fact is the root cause of fear. Fear can only exist in a state of unawareness. In a state of full consciousness, **fear cannot exist.**

HAPPINESS AND FEARLESSNESS

ITS ORIGIN AND THE PHYSICAL EFFECTS

From the psychological point of view, emotional conduct and behaviour rise from the hypothalamus—that part of the brain which makes up the floor and part of the lateral walls of the third ventricle. There are such centres in our body where different kinds of inclination flow. Passions flow from the body. All emotions have their origin in the hypothalamus, which is the centre of fear.

The doctrine of karma postulates unconsciousness as the stimulator of fear. It is ignorance which gives rise to fear. Among the various states of unconsciousness, one is fear. It is because of fear that man cannot perceive reality.

There are different gestures for every feeling, every sentiment. Thought, feeling and gesture are linked to one another. Our facial gestures are determined by inner feelings. Fear expresses itself in a way peculiar to itself. The face of a man in the grip of fear shrinks. Likewise, the body. Both the body and the face shrink and expand. Fear contracts while joy expands. Irradiated by joy, the face opens up like a flower. On the other hand, the face of a frightened person shrinks. It appears quite emaciated. Changes wrought by fear in the outer appearance are quite apparent. However, the inner parts of the body also manifest these changes. The heart beats faster, the blood pressure goes high, the throat dries up, the glands secreting saliva are deactivated, the face becomes lean, the stomach and the intestines contract, and there is a loss of appetite. A man who lives constantly in a state of fear has little appetite. The conductivity of the skin stands altered; it grows hypersensitive.

A man commits a crime. When presented before the judge, the man, afraid of getting exposed, lies and claims that he is innocent. But how is the judge to establish that the man is a liar? That he is a criminal? Of late, certain devices, like the galvanometer, have been created. The machine is switched on and the man is made to stand before it. The man is afraid of getting caught. This fear gives rise to excitement. His inner being gets disturbed. The moving hand of the galvanometer indicates the disturbance, and conclusively establishes that the man is not at ease, and that is because he has lied. A device like the galvanometer thus establishes the truth. All this happens through the conductivity of the skin which is measured by the galvanometer and which gives us the truth. In a fit of rage or fear or any other strong emotions, both the outward appearance and the inward state undergo a change and this change reveals the truth. A man assumes a thousand poses during the course of a single day. With the help of a sensitive, high-frequency camera, these varying positions can be photographed and the difference between one pose and another can be established clearly. The pose of five minutes ago is completely different from the pose five minutes later. As the inner feelings change, there is a corresponding change in a man's countenance. Even the science of face-reading is based upon that. On the basis of the shape and structure of the face, a man's proclivities, and even his future, can be foretold.

Fear is a strong emotion. A man's countenance in a state of fear shows distress and is strangely disturbing. Whosoever comes in contact with a fear-oppressed man soon imbibes his restlessness. How does it pass on? The visitor would not know why, but he would be disquieted.

When the feeling of fearlessness is awakened in a person, it shows itself in his features. The outward proof of the absence of fear is gaiety; the face blossoms. There is deep tranquillity from within. There is perfect joy. When the current of fearlessness flows, the sympathetic nervous system becomes active. There is no turbulence anywhere. One experiences profound peace and joy. It feels good to be alive.

THE HIGHWAY TO FEARLESSNESS

The question arises: How can we live largely in a state of fearlessness? How can we ensure a ceaseless current of fearlessness? How do we experience a state of fearlessness? Any kind of fear is harmful; while fearlessness is beneficial. We must abandon the stream of fear and enter the stream of fearlessness. For this the right techniques and the right means are necessary.

CHARACTER AND CONDUCT

There is a path leading to fearlessness. This relates to our character and conduct. Fear springs from violence, untruth, and total acquisitiveness. These are the three great causes intimately connected with our character. Every man knows what creates acquisitiveness—fear. A man leaves his house but, mid-way, he remembers that he has forgotten to lock it. He returns immediately, fearful lest some thief get in. Why this fear? It is because he is so attached to the things which he has accumulated that he cannot look with equanimity upon the prospect of being deprived of them. There are many people who do not even make use of their accumulations. At the time of making yearly accounts on the occasion of Diwali or Ramnavmi, they calculate what profits they have made, their wealth and how much their wealth has increased, and the very thought of it gives them deep satisfaction as nothing else in the world can. The mere realization that 'I have so much!' is highly gratifying. Apart from the vast accumulation made, their wealth has no meaning and no utility; it is never consumed. But the very fact of possession makes them so happy that it becomes their summum bonum in life. And yet, this realization creates such fear that they know no rest all day and night. They are afraid of being cheated and are tormented by fear. They find a great psychological satisfaction in possession, but this is forever accompanied by the fear that, one day, they may be cheated of their possessions. Gratification is momentary but the fear is constant. Accumulation leads to the greatest fear.

Untruth is also a great cause of fear. A man may thoughtlessly tell a lie but is constantly possessed by the fear of getting exposed.

Violence, too, is born of fear. As long a man is possessed by violence, untruth and acquisitiveness, fearlessness cannot be an intrinsic quality of his character.

What really works is the strength of one's character. When a man's character develops the state of fearlessness, total freedom from fear gradually comes into being. The state inherent in fearlessness does wonders. Whatever a man does then is right. The greatest obstacles that a man faces in the fulfilment of his tasks are fear, mistrust and suspicion. When a man embarks upon a new venture, he is immediately assailed by doubts. 'Will I succeed or not?' he asks himself. 'If I fail, what will people say?' How can a man afflicted with such fear and mistrust really succeed?

The great secret of success is the development of character. The three great pillars of character development are non-violence, truth and non-acquisitiveness.

If we want to enter the state of fearlessness, we must develop in ourselves the spirit of non-violence, for it is one aspect of fearlessness. We must also pursue truth, for truth is another aspect of fearlessness and, with it, we must also cultivate non-acquisitiveness, the third aspect of fearlessness. A man in whose heart these feelings dwell is bound to enter the state of fearlessness.

We are surprised when told that Lord Mahavira was bitten by a ferocious snake named Chandkaushik and yet he remained unmoved. There is, however, nothing unusual in the occurrence. If the snake had bitten any Tom, Dick or Harry and if the man had stayed unperturbed, it certainly would have been surprising. But for a man like Mahavira, who was constantly and fully aware of himself, the poison of a snake, or of a scorpion, was quite immaterial. A man who has reached the highest ground of spirituality is not disturbed by a snake or its poison, and the poison, however dangerous, wouldn't have any adverse effect on him.

The experience of complete consciousness is the experience of the state of fearlessness. Likewise the experience of bliss. We are not talking of pleasure or joy, but of real happiness. Fear is always inherent in pleasure. Joy and sorrow are linked together. Every joy is followed by sorrow, as every sorrow is followed by joy; they make an inseparable pair.

FEARLESSNESS THROUGH ANUPREKSHA

One of the techniques for developing fearlessness is anupreksha (contemplation). Through it, it is possible to develop the flow of fearlessness. Within our body there lie many systems of vibrations. The paths, the tracks and the highways are all there, by means of which sound vibrations pervade the entire organism, and influence our conduct. The ancient doctrine of vibrations is very comprehensive. This doctrine was well established about three thousand years ago, long before the development of the quantum theory. According to it, the world is nothing but a series of vibrations, wave after wave of sensation. A wave of fear arises and, immediately, vibrations of fear overwhelm the earth and the sky. If, at that very point in time, we could somehow start a wave of fearlessness, if we could produce vibrations of fearlessness, the wave of fear would be dissolved. The doctrine of anupreksha is a contralateral doctrine which lays down that one wave can transcend another, that if a good wave can be started, the bad one would be rendered ineffective. Similarly, a bad wave, if stronger than the good one, would destroy it. Our valour, intelligence and vision determine what we will do at a particular time, and what kind of effort we will put in. A man who has practised preksha meditation, one who has perceived the truth that an evil wave can be countermanded by a good one, that a negative wave can be supplanted by a positive one, becomes alert, so that as soon as an evil thought arises in his mind, he sets about releasing a counter wave of goodness that would repel the former.

FEARLESSNESS THROUGH PREKSHA DHYANA

Another means of attaining the state of fearlessness is preksha. With the gradual development of the power of seeing, our perception becomes truth-oriented. Whatever fear there is, it is because of untruth. False belief, false doctrine, false conception, and false determination—whatever the aspect of untruth, it only creates fear. As our vision develops, we perceive the truth more clearly. We bid goodbye to fiction. We grow stronger, and fear decreases. There is no fear in facing a fact, but fear is inherent in illusion, in the state of unconsciousness, and in untruth. Preksha becomes the means of breaking the cycle of ignorance, and when this cycle breaks, fear is dissolved.

Preksha, anupreksha, and the repetition of mantra—these techniques were developed primarily for the evolution of fearlessness.

FEARLESSNESS THROUGH MANTRAS

In every tradition—Jain, Buddhist or Vedic—there exist mantras for the prevention of fear. Some people get frightened in their sleep; they have terrifying dreams at night. Others get frightened for no cause. In order to avoid such predicaments, hundreds of mantras have been evolved and they have been used to good effect. They help divert attention from fear. The very condition of the mind gets altered. Also, a great many remedies have been evolved. There are many medicines, roots and herbs which, if placed beside the pillow, stop fear altogether. All dreams cease. The roots and herbs and the mantras have been useful, and research in this direction has yielded good results.

There may be a brief interval between joy and sorrow but, sooner or later, one is bound to be followed by the other. But bliss is beyond pleasure and pain, beyond joy and sorrow. Preksha gives rise to waves of bliss—that bliss which is allied with equanimity. In equanimity, there is bliss. In that state, there is total freedom from fear.

ESSENCE

- Happiness is beyond joy and sorrow.
- Complete absence of fear and happiness go together.
- Fear is the outcome of negative thinking.
- The experience of complete consciousness is the experience of the state of fearlessness.

CONTEMPLATION OF FEARLESSNESS

1. **POSTURE:**
   Select a posture in which you can sit comfortably and continuously for forty-five minutes—full lotus, half lotus, cross-legged or diamond.

2. **MUDRAS—THE POSITION OF THE HANDS (ANY ONE):**
   i. Gyana Mudra:
      Place your right hand on the right knee and the left on the left knee, palms turned up. Touch the tip of the thumb with the tip of the index finger with a slight pressure. Keep the other fingers straight and relaxed.
   ii. Brahma Mudra:
      Place both hands on your lap, one above the other, palms turned up, the left palm under the right one. Keep your eyes softly closed.

3. **RECITATION OF MAHAPRANA DHVANI:**
   - Keep your lips softly closed, your spinal column and neck straight, without stiffness.
   - Inhale deeply and silently for about four to five

seconds with a calm mind, empty of thoughts, all muscles relaxed.
- Concentrate on the top of your head.
- Keeping your lips closed, exhale slowly, making the sound of mmm .... through the nostrils, like the buzzing of a bee.
- This may last eight to ten seconds. Inhale again and keep repeating this exercise for five minutes.

4. KAYOTSARGA (RELAXATION)
- Relax all the muscles in your body.
- Release all the stress from your body.
- Concentrate and allow your mind to travel, taking a trip to all the parts of your body, from the big toe of your right foot to the top of the head.
- Give an auto-suggestion to each and every muscle to relax and feel it relaxing.
- Concentrate deeply and remain completely alert.

5. With your mind's eye, visualize that everything around you—including the air itself—is coloured a bright rosy pink.

Take a deep breath and, as you slowly inhale, visualize that you are breathing in a long stream of bright pink air. Repeat the breathing exercise several times, each time inhaling bright pink air. Visualize that bright pink air entering your lungs with each inhalation.

6. Concentrate your full attention on the centre of bliss situated near the heart and loudly recite nine times:
   'My fearlessness is increasing.
   My feeling of fear is diminishing.'
   Now, repeat the same sentences mentally nine times:
   'My fearlessness is increasing.
   My feeling of fear is diminishing.'

7. Contemplate the high moral value of this virtue in the following lines:
   'Fear withers even the developed abilities and does not permit the latent ones to be developed. I must, therefore, strive to attain the virtue of fearlessness.
   Everybody tries to frighten the one who is afraid. Fear makes one a coward.
   A coward attracts neither respect nor sympathy. I firmly resolve to attain fearlessness in order to develop my latent inner strength.
   Undoubtedly, I will attain freedom from fear.'

Conclude the meditation session by chanting the mahaprana dhvani three times.